Role of Imaging in Adults with Congenital Heart Disease: State-of-Art Review

DEDICATION

To my wife Karma and our son Adnan,
Thank you for your support while writing this book.

CONTENTS

FOREWORD

The success of congenital heart surgery is evident in any general cardiology practice today. Young, and sometimes not so young, adults with repaired or palliated cardiac birth defects are routinely observed in ever increasing numbers in general adult practice, which is a testament to the nearly seven decades of success and progress in the childhood care of these patients by pediatric cardiologists and congenital heart surgeons. More than 85% of infants born with congenital heart disease (CHD) can be expected to survive to reach adulthood, and that statistic, based on the less-developed surgical practices of the era in which these adults were first treated, will continue to improve as techniques.

The challenges remain considerable and the care of surviving and often thriving adult CHD patients has been the focus of several comprehensive guidelines, including AHA/ACC 2008 Guidelines for the Management of Adults With Congenital Heart Disease. But, true to Korzybski's saying "the map is not the territory," the wordy guidelines are not the patient, nor the patient's plan of evaluation and treatment.

Not coincidentally, the last few decades of success in the treatment of CHD has been paralleled by fantastic advances in diagnostic imaging. This has not only proved to be of great benefit, but also a tremendous challenge, to those of us not trained as radiologists. The role of imaging is a key in the follow-up and timely intervention of adult CHD patients who often bear a subclinical burden of postoperative pathology into their adult years, and in whom presymptomatic recognition of trouble is frequently needed.

My colleagues, Dr's. AlJaroudi, McLarry, Lloyd, and Iskandrian, have done a great service to adult CHD patients with the publication of The Role of Imaging in Adults with Congenital Heart Disease: State-of-the-Art Review. It serves as more than a guide, and considerably more than a map, in navigating the often arcane world of adult CHD cardiovascular anatomy. This book is textually succinct, exactly what one would expect in a work containing highly clear and informative illustrations of cutting edge cardiovascular imaging. This work brings us much closer to finding our way through the bewildering territory where we often find our patients lost within, and I recommend it to the readers as an office and bedside companion to other essential items, including the guidelines, and consultation with congenital heart disease specialists.

Walter H. Johnson, Jr., ***M.D., FACC***
University of Alabama at Birmingham
Birmingham, Alabama
USA

PREFACE

This book is intended to serve as a reference to help clinicians understand the role, advantages and limitations of the different imaging modalities (echocardiography, CT, MRI, nuclear, and catheterization) in the diagnosis, follow-up and clinical care of adult patients with congenital heart disease.

This book is different in the respect that it is written for the general cardiologist in a simplified way. It is a summary of the guidelines and up-to-date studies on the different imaging modalities used in congenital heart disease. The book is divided into four sections; shunt lesions, left-sided obstructive lesions, cyanotic lesions, and other congenital cardiac lesions. It covers the most common types encountered in practice.

Wael AlJaroudi, *MD*
University of Alabama at Birmingham,
Birmingham, AL
USA

CONTRIBUTORS LIST

Wael AlJaroudi, MD
Division of Cardiovascular Disease,
Department of lnternal Medicine,
University of Alabama at Birmingham,
Birmingham, AL

Joel McLarry, MD
Departments of Internal Medicine and Pediatrics,
University of Alabama at Birmingham,
Birmingham, AL

Steve Lloyd, MD, FACC
Division of Cardiovascular Disease,
Department of lnternal Medicine,
University of Alabama at Birmingham,
Birmingham, AL

Ami E. Iskandrian, MD, MACC
Division of Cardiovascular Disease,
Department of lnternal Medicine,
University of Alabama at Birmingham,
Birmingham, AL

ABBREVIATIONS

2DE: Two- dimensional echocardiography

3DE: Three-dimensional echocardiography

AS: Aortic stenosis

ASD: Atrial septal defect

AV: Aortic valve

CC: Cardiac catheterization

CHD: Congenital heart disease

CT: Computed tomography

ECG: Electrocardiogram

HF: Heart failure

LV: Left ventricle/ventricular

MR: Magnetic resonance imaging

PDA: Patent ductus arteriosus

PHT: Pulmonary hypertension

PS: Pulmonic stenosis

Qp: Pulmonary blood flow

Qs: Systemic blood flow

RNA: Radionuclide angiography

RV: Right ventricle/ventricular

TEE: Transesophageal echocardiography

TGA: Transposition of the Great Arteries

TTE: Transthoracic echocardiography

VSD: Ventricular septal defect

INTRODUCTION

Approximately 40,000 infants are born each year with a congenital heart disease (CHD) in the United States. CHD is defined as any abnormality that affects the cardiac anatomy or physiology, with some forms manifesting at birth, or during infancy, as cyanosis, failure to thrive, or heart failure (HF), while others are discovered in adulthood or incidentally. Newer imaging modalities, improved surgical techniques and medical care, have increased the survival rate of these patients [1]. In the year 2000, it was estimated that there were 485,000 adults with complex CHD and 300,000 with simple CHD in the United States [2]; these numbers have been increasing exponentially over the years. As these patients grow older, they may develop arrhythmias, HF, shunts, conduit failures, valvular insufficiency, and pulmonary hypertension (PHT). In addition, they are 25-100 times more likely to experience sudden cardiac death than the general population [3]. Also, adult women with surgically repaired complex CHD often encounter additional problems during pregnancy.

Evaluating a patient with CHD is challenging since these lesions are diverse and can be complex. For a full evaluation, it is important to identify the type of CHD, the morphological and physiological chambers, anomalous structures, persistent shunts, ventricular function, valvular stenosis or regurgitation, and assess the degree of PHT. Various modalities are needed to make these assessments depending on the nature of the heart pathology (Table **1**).

Table 1. Applications of Various Imaging Modalities in Congenital Heart Diseases in Adults

Structures	Most common imaging modalities used
1. LV function	TTE, 3DE, Nuclear, MRI, CT, CC
2. RV function	TTE, 3DE, Nuclear, MRI, CT, CC
3. Pulmonary hypertension	TTE, MRI, CC
4. Shunt detection/quantification	TTE, 3DE, TEE, MRI, CC, Nuclear
5. Defects/anomalous structures	TTE, 3DE, TEE, MRI, CT. CC
6. Anomalous coronary arteries	TEE, MRI, CT, CC
7. Myocardial ischemia/scar	TTE, Nuclear, MRI, CT, stress Echo

Abbreviations: 3DE: 3D echocardiography, CC: cardiac catheterization, CT: computed tomography, LV: left ventricle, TEE: transesophageal echocardiogram, MRI: magnetic resonance imaging, RV: right ventricle.

The most common types of adult CHD during the time period 2002 to 2008, based on the Concor registry, are shown in Figure **1** [4]. The purpose of this review is to examine the relative merits of different imaging modalities in relation to adult CHD.

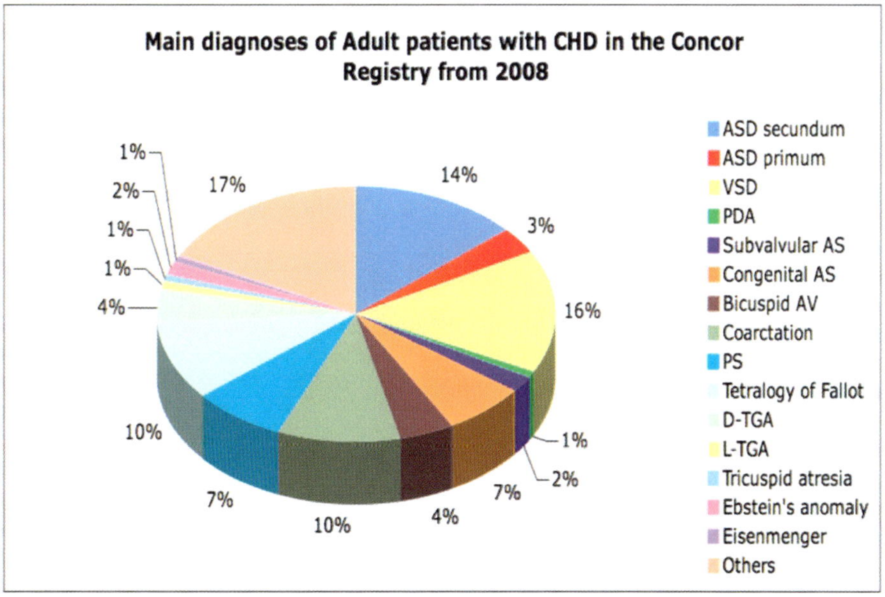

Figure 1. Most common types of adult congenital heart diseases. [Modified from Reference 4].

CHAPTER I

Shunt Lesions

Wael AlJaroudi[*,1], Steve Lloyd[1], Ami E. Iskandrian[1] and Joel McLarry[2]

[1]*Division of Cardiovascular Disease, Department of Internal Medicine, University of Alabama at Birmingham, Birmingham, AL, USA*

[2]*Departments of Internal Medicine and Pediatrics, University of Alabama at Birmingham, Birmingham, AL, USA*

Abstract: Detection of intracardiac shunts is imperative to prevent paradoxical thromboembolism and heart strain from a shunt's additional flow. Multiple modalities are used to detect shunts, including echocardiography, MRI, CC, and nuclear modalities. Echocardiography is the initial imaging modality for ASD, VSD, and PDA. In ASD and VSD, TEE, 3DE and MRI play a complementary role and can help to determine the suitability for percutaneous closure. Percutaneous closure is being increasingly used for ASD and PDA repair, while percutaneous VSD repair still remains in the experimental stage.

1. SHUNT DETECTION AND QUANTIFICATION

Intra-cardiac shunts place patients at risk for paradoxical thromboembolism in addition to exerting stress on the cardiac chambers. Quantification of shunts is necessary for clinical decision making since it can help determine the appropriateness and urgency of shunt repair. Table **2** lists several studies that quantitated intra-cardiac shunts using multiple imaging modalities [5-19].

Table 2. Shunt Quantifications Using Different Imaging Modalities

Imaging Modality	Year	Type of Shunt	N	Correlation with CC	Refs.
Echocardiography	1998	ASD	32	0.93	5
	2001	VSD	30	0.86	6
	2002	ASD	22	0.86	7
	2004	ASD	46	0.98	8
	2005	ASD,VSD	120	0.82-0.96	9
MRI	1992	ASD	11	0.91	10
	1995	ASD,VSD,PDA	11	0.94	11
	2002	ASD,VSD,PDA	17	0.91	12
	2006	ASD	22	0.95	13
	2006	VSD	14	0.90	14
Nuclear	1976	ASD/VSD	105	0.94	15
	1981	ASD/VSD/PDA	38	0.84	16
	1982	ASD	16	0.81	17
	1982	ASD/VSD/PDA	15	0.79	18
	1984	ASD/VSD	65	0.76	19

Abbreviations: ASD (atrial septal defect), CC (cardiac catheterization), MRI (magnetic resonance imaging), N (number of patients), PDA (patent ductus arteriosus), VSD (ventricular septal defect) [5-19].

*Corresponding Author: 701 19th Street, LHRB 306, Birmingham, AL 35294-0007, Alabama, USA; Tel: 205-934-0820; Fax: 205-934-7579; E-mail: wjaroudi@hotmail.com

Wael AlJaroudi (Ed.)

Oximetry is the most commonly used method during cardiac catheterization (CC) to detect and quantify intra-cardiac shunts. It has been dubbed as the "gold standard" in most studies. The main limitations of oximetry are its utilization of invasive techniques, the lack of a steady state between sample collections, and its low sensitivity in small shunts. In addition, in patent ductus arteriosus (PDA), the oxygen saturation from the main or right pulmonary artery is lower than the left pulmonary artery because of preferential shunting which could introduce significant errors unless suspected. The indocyanine green-dye dilution and intracardiac ECG recording during hydrogen inhalation are other methods that are available to invasively quantitate shunts; The dye-dilution is a quantitative method, while the platinum tip catheter (used in conjunction with hydrogen inhalation) is a qualitative method and is therefore seldom used. Contrast angiography has been used to detect and quantify shunts as well [20].

Two-dimensional echocardiography (2DE) and Doppler currently are the most widely used methods to quantify and detect intra-cardiac shunts. The shunt is determined as the ratio of pulmonary (Qp) to systemic (Qs) blood flow: Qp/Qs = (Right ventricular [RV] outflow tract area x RV outflow tract velocity time integral)/ (Left ventricular [LV] outflow tract area x LV outflow velocity time integral) [21]. These calculations are based on the assumptions that flow occurs in a rigid tube at a constant velocity and that the outflow tract is cylindrical in shape with a constant cross sectional area throughout the cardiac cycle; these assumptions may not always be true. Additional limitations include errors in measurement from inappropriate beam alignment, and errors in outflow diameter measurements [21, 22]. Shunt fraction can also be determined as the ratio of RV stroke volume/LV stroke volume. This method, however, is not accurate in patients with valvular regurgitation or with ventricular septal defects (VSD) [21, 22]. Saline contrast echocardiography also plays a role in shunt detection, identifying ASDs, VSDs, and post-operative baffle leaks in Senning and Mustard operations [23]. Furthermore, saline contrast is also useful for the detection of pulmonary arteriovenous shunting in cavopulmonary anastomosis, such as in Glenn and Fontan circulations [24]. However, despite the utility of these modalities, right heart enlargement often serves as a surrogate marker for significant left-to-right shunts and most clinical decisions for intracardiac shunt closure rely on this.

Velocity encoding magnetic resonance imaging (MRI) allows calculation of flow through the aortic and pulmonary valves. MRI is also excellent for assessment for extracardiac structures especially in coarctation of the aorta, anomalous pulmonary venous return and heterotaxy. However, turbulent jet, velocity aliasing, motion or breathing artifacts, off-axis through plane and the presence of indwelling devices (pacemakers, AICDs) are some of its limitations. Stroke volumes can also be used to determine shunt ratios in a manner similar to 2DE. The major drawback is valvular regurgitation or VSD that make such calculations less accurate [25].

Radionuclide angiography (RNA), either gated equilibrium or first-pass, has also been used in the past for this indication [26]. The equilibrium method measures the RV and LV stroke volumes and shunt fraction. Similar to 2DE and MRI, valvular regurgitation is a major source of error. The first-pass method is similar in principle to the dye-dilution method used during CC. Its major limitations include disintegration of the bolus because of poor injection, large right atrium, dilated RV, tricuspid and pulmonary regurgitations, and PHT [26]. Currently RNA is seldom used to quantitate shunts.

2. ATRIAL SEPTAL DEFECT (ASD)

ASD is the most common CHD in adults (Figure **1**). Although the diagnosis is often made in infancy, it can go undetected until much later in adult life. The three most common types are secundum (70%), primum (20%), sinus venosus (10%), and, the uncommon, coronary sinus defect (<1%). Approximately 10% of secundum and 90-100% of sinus venosus ASDs are associated with anomalous pulmonary venous drainage to the right atrium [27]. The primum type is commonly associated with cleft mitral valve, subvalvular aortic stenosis and/or mitral valve prolapse.

If uncorrected, arrhythmias, HF, and Eisenmenger physiology can occur. Imaging helps define the size, shape and location of the defect, degree of shunting, LV/RV function, the presence of anomalous pulmonary veins, degree of PHT, and suitability for percutaneous closure.

Role of Imaging

M-Mode echocardiography typically shows RV enlargement and paradoxical interventricular septal movement. Although these may be non-specific findings, they do alert the reader to the possibility of a significant left-to-right shunt as a result of the ASD. Transthoracic 2DE (TTE) on the other hand, shows a discontinuity of the interatrial septal membrane and enlargement of the right chambers. Color Doppler shows flow through the defect [21]. The sensitivity and specificity in detecting an ASD and associated anomalous pulmonary veins are listed in Table **3** [28-38].

The TTE is very sensitive in visualizing ASD secundum; the right parasternal approach and injection of agitated saline increase the sensitivity [29] while severe PHT and poor acoustic window decrease it [29,37-40]. However, TTE often misses anomalous pulmonary veins and sinus venosus defects (see Table **3**). In this setting, transesophageal echocardiography (TEE) is advantageous with a higher sensitivity (>90%). There are limited data regarding the sensitivity of transthoracic 3DE in detecting ASD. Marx *et al.* found a sensitivity of 81% using old-generation equipment [41]. The advantage of 3DE, however, is that it offers an en face view of the defect with information about the aortic rim tissue, which is invaluable when considering percutaneous closure.

Table 3. Sensitivity and Specificity of Imaging Modalities in the Diagnosis of Shunt Lesions in Adults

CHD	Imaging modality	N	Sensitivity	Specificity	Refs.
ASD secundum	TTE	93,20	89-95%	90-100%	28,29
	TEE	120	100%	100%	30
	MRI	31	100%	100%	31
Sinus Venosus	TTE	16	44%	100%	28
	TEE	25,62	100%	100%	32,33
	MRI	16	95-100%	100%	34
Anomalous pulmonary veins	TTE	25	10-38%	-	32
	TEE	25,62	81-96%	100%	32,33
	MRI	16	95-100%	100%	34
ASD primum	TTE	32	100%	100%	28
	TEE	8	100%	100%	29
	MRI	31,16	86-98%	100%	31,34
VSD (all types)	TTE	50	74%	100%	35
	TEE	62	92%	92%	33
	MRI	26	95-100%	90-100%	36
PDA	TTE	40	12-50%	100%	37
	TEE	40	97-100%	100%	37
	MRI	49	94%	95%	38

Abbreviations: ASD: atrial septum defect, MRI: magnetic resonance imaging, TEE: transesophageal echocardiography, TTE: transthoracic echocardiography, VSD: ventricular septum defect, PDA: patent ductus arteriosus

The size and shape of the ASD correlate with the magnitude of shunting and determine the suitability for percutaneous closure. Table **4** lists the major studies used to determine the size of the ASD [6,42-54]. The measurements correlate well with the balloon diameter used during CC (r=0.76-0.98). The appropriateness of echocardiography in ASD is outlined in table 5 [55,56].

Percutaneous closure of ASD has become increasingly popular over the last few years. Common indications for closure are listed in table 6 [57]. The presence of anomalous pulmonary veins, deficient rims in more than one quadrant, a defect size > 35-40 mm, and severe PHT preclude percutaneous repair. The largest series in this regard is from 2001 (3580 patients) in which the procedures were guided by TEE with a 97% success rate and <0.3% major complications [59]. Intra-cardiac echocardiography guided closure (Figure **2a**) has recently become popular with similar success and complication rates [45,49,60]. Potential complications include atrial arrhythmias (<4%), device embolization (<2%), residual shunt (<4%), size mismatch (<5%), vascular access problem, device erosion and cardiac tamponade (<0.1%) [61]. Intra-cardiac echocardio-graphy-assisted percutaneous ASD closure is performed without the use of conscious sedation; it offers accurate information, and detects additional findings missed by TTE and TEE in up to one third of patients [60].

Table 4. Role of Imaging in Determining the Size of the ASD and VSD

CHD	Imaging Modality	Year	N	Method	Gold Standard(s)	Correlation coefficient	Refs.
ASD	Echo	1988	23	2D TTE	CC	0.57	40
		1997	34	3D TTE	MRI/Surgery	0.97/0.95	41
		2000	39	3D TEE	Balloon diameter	0.98	42
		2001	30	2D TTE	Balloon diameter	0.80-0.84	6
		2003	82	ICE	Balloon diameter	No difference	43
		2004	12	3D TTE	Balloon diameter	No difference	44
		2004	66	2D TEE	Balloon diameter	0.76	45
		2006	30	2D TEE	Balloon diameter	0.89	46
		2006	29	3D TTE	Balloon diameter	0.92	46
		2007	14	ICE	TEE	No difference	47
	MRI	1995	30	Phase contrast	Balloon diameter	0.93	48
		2004	66	Phase contrast	Balloon diameter	0.78	45
		2008	44	SSFP	Balloon diameter	0.80	49
		2008	60	SSFP	Balloon diameter	0.77	50
VSD	Echo	2004	38	3D TTE	Surgery	0.92	46
		2004	38	2D TTE	Surgery	0.69	46
		2005	12	2D TTE/ICE	Balloon diameter	No difference	51
		2006	34	3D TTE	Surgery	0.95	52
	MRI	-	-	-	-	-	-

Abbreviations as in tables 1-3.

Table 5. Appropriateness Score for Transthoracic, Transesophageal, CT, and MRI in the Diagnosis of Adults with Congenital Heart Diseases

	Appropriateness score (1-9)		
CHD	**TTE/TEE**	**CT**	**MRI**
Simple CHD (ASD, VSD, PDA)	A (9)	I (3)	U (5)
Anomalous pulmonary veins	A (9)	A (7)	A (8)
Congenital valvular stenosis	A (9)	U (5)	U (5)
Complex CHD	A (9)	A (7)	A (9)
Anomalies of the great vessels	A (9)	A (7)	A (9)
Anomalous coronary arteries	U (5)	A (7)	A (9)

Abbreviations as in tables 1-4.
ACC appropriateness criteria: A (score 7-9): Appropriate; U (score 4-6): Uncertain; I (score 1-3): Inappropriate. [Modified from references 55 and 56].

With MRI, the image quality is not affected by body habitus, imaging can be performed in any plane (Figure **2b**), and anomalous pulmonary veins (Figure **2c**) and other defects can be visualized in almost all cases [34]. MRI could determine the shunt and size of the ASD (see Tables **2** and **4**). In the study by Thomson *et al*, MRI identified extra findings that altered the clinical decision in up to 20% of the patients, including insufficient rim tissue, anomalous pulmonary veins, and multiple defects [51]. Imaging time is longer with MRI than TTE, requires breath-holding and patient cooperation, and is not readily available in all centers. Cardiac CT and nuclear imaging are not used at present to diagnose ASD.

Recommendation

Imaging in a patient with suspected ASD should start with TTE, which is inexpensive, fast, and readily available. The use of the right parasternal approach, agitated saline and Doppler improve the accuracy. TEE provides more accurate information on the size and shape of the defect and its suitability for percutaneous closure. If a sinus venosus defect or anomalous pulmonary veins are suspected but not visualized, TEE, 3DE or MRI may be performed. At present, 3DE, TEE, and intra-cardiac echocardiography are used to guide percutaneous closure.

3. VENTRICULAR SEPTAL DEFECT (VSD)

VSD is the second most common adult CHD. VSDs can be associated with ASD (35%), PDA (22%), right aortic arch (13%), and aortic regurgitation. The most common types are membranous (75-80%); muscular (5-20%); inlet (8%); and outlet (5-7%) [61]. If untreated, HF and PHT develop. The role of imaging is to identify the defect location, size and shape, degree of shunt, LV/RV function, PHT, and suitability for closure.

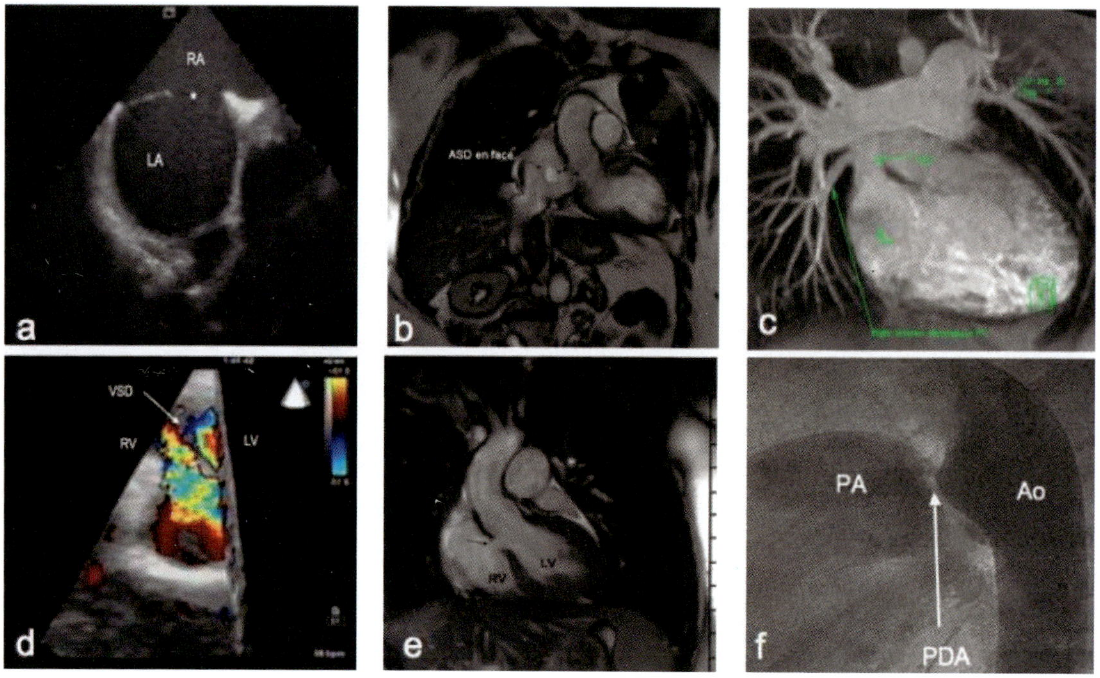

Figure 2. Various types of shunt lesions

a. Intra-cardiac echocardiogram shows an atrial septal defect (asterix) prior to percutaneous closure.

b. MRI en face view demonstrates an atrial septal defect with surrounding aortic rim tissue. Noted is the close proximity of the defect to the aorta.

c. MRI view of a right anomalous inferior pulmonary vein draining into the SVC in a patient with a sinus venosus defect.

d. 3DE with color Doppler showing a VSD and flow between the left and right ventricles.

e. MRI showing a peri-membranous VSD (arrow).

f. Contrast angiogram showing flow from the aorta to the pulmonary artery through the PDA.

Role of Imaging

TTE with Doppler is the non-invasive method of choice (see Table **5**). It has a sensitivity of 88-95% and a specificity of 99% (see Table **3**). VSDs <5mm in diameter and apical muscular defects are difficult to detect [62]. Also, severe PHT and poor acoustic window lower the sensitivity, while imaging in multiple planes and using Doppler increase the sensitivity [39,61]; 3DE and TEE are used as adjuncts whenever there is uncertainty.

In most cases, with the caveats cited above, TTE accurately determines the size of the defect (see Table **5**); 3DE provides en face view of the defect and adjacent structures (Figure **2d**) while TEE overcomes the limitation of poor acoustic window and therefore its findings correlate better with surgical measurements.

Doppler measures the velocity of the tricuspid regurgitation jet and provides a good estimate of PHT. The presence of RV hypertrophy, chamber enlargement, and interventricular septal wall flattening in diastole and systole suggest PHT. The absence of tricuspid regurgitation, eccentric or torrential TR jet, might underestimate the degree of PHT [21].

Percutaneous VSD closure has been performed more frequently in recent years (see Table **6**), but still remains largely investigational. However, patients with a hemodynamically significant shunt, a favorable defect size (4-18 mm), shape, location (> 2 mm tissue rim from the aortic valve), and without severe PHT are candidates for this procedure [57]. Intra-cardiac or TEE assisted percutaneous VSD closure is successful in 96%-98% of patients with 1.0-2.8 % major complication rate(atrio-ventricular block, embolization, perforation, valvular regurgitation, arrhythmias, and hemolysis) and a 0.5% death rate [53, 63-64].

Table 6. Indications and Level of Evidence for the Common Percutaneous Interventions in Adults with Congenital Heart Diseases

	Intervention	Indication	Level of evidence
ASD	Closure	RA or RV overload	I:B
		Orthodeoxia-platypnea	IIa:B
VSD	Closure	LV overload, Qp/Qs >2	I:B
		Qp/Qs >1.5, PA pressure <2/3 systemic	IIa:B
		History of infective endocarditis	I:C
PDA	Closure	Heart failure, severe PHT	I:B
		Asymptomatic with audible murmur	IIb:B
AS	Valvuloplasty	Asymptomatic, peak gradient > 60 mm Hg	I:B
		Symptomatic, peak gradient >50 mm Hg	I:B
Coarctation of the aorta	Dilation	≥20 mm Hg peak gradient	I:C
		<20mm Hg gradient with significant collateral flow	I:C
PVS	Valvuloplasty	Asymptomatic, mean gradient >40 mm Hg	I:B
		Symptomatic, mean gradient >30 mm Hg, RV dysfunction	I:B
PAS	Angioplasty	> 50% diameter narrowing, an elevated RV systolic pressure >50 mm Hg, and/or symptoms.	I:B
		RV pressure >50% systemic levels	IIa:B
Conduit/Baffle stenosis	Dilation	RV pressure >50% systemic	IIa:B
		RV pressure >25% systemic with cyanosis, severe pulmonary regurgitation, or RV dysfunction	IIa:B

Abbreviations: AI: aortic insufficiency, AS: aortic stenosis, PAS: pulmonary artery stenosis, PHT: pulmonary hypertension, PS: pulmonary valve stenosis, Other abbreviations as in tables 1-5
Level of evidence is based on the ACC format. [Modified from reference 57, 58]

MRI has a limited role in evaluating isolated VSDs, though it might prove helpful in detecting apical or multiple VSDs in complex CHD (see Table **5**) (Figure **2e**). CT and nuclear imaging are not used at present and when CC is used, cine ventriculography can aid VSD visualization especially when performed in the left anterior oblique projection.

Recommendation

TTE with Doppler should be the first imaging modality to diagnose VSD. 3DE can help determine suitability for percutaneous repair. Alternatively, TEE or MRI may be used if the acoustic window is poor and/or the VSD is complex.

4. PATENT DUCTUS ARTERIOSUS (PDA)

PDA is a congenital defect that represents failure of the ductus to close after birth. It is may be seen concomitantly with ASDs and VSDs. If untreated, potential complications include HF, PHT, and, rarely, endarteritis.

Role of Imaging

M-mode echocardiography demonstrates left atrial and LV enlargement, which are non-specific findings [39]. TTE with Doppler is sensitive in children or young patients with good acoustic windows, showing diastolic ductal flow into the pulmonary artery. However, acoustic shadowing in adults lowers the sensitivity to 42%, while severe PHT reduces it further to 12% [37] (see Table **3**). Pulmonary insufficiency, aorto-pulmonary defects, or coronary artery fistula may cause false-positive results and lower the specificity of TTE [37, 40]. TEE does not have these limitations and can diagnose PDA with 97% sensitivity. Furthermore, TEE is more accurate in detecting PDAs in patients with Eisenmenger syndrome [37].

Although a PDA must be large to be visualized by MRI, detection of the flow void caused by turbulent flow passing through the defect into the pulmonary artery is a sensitive and reliable method to diagnose PDA [36] (see Table **3**). MRI is currently not considered an initial imaging option to diagnose PDA (Table **5**). CT and nuclear modalities have limited role in the evaluation of PDA as well. The main role of CC (Figure **2f**) is in percutaneous device closure (see Table **6**); the choice of the device (coil, Amplatzer or others) depends on the size and length of the defect, which is accurately determined during the procedure. The success rate of percutaneous repair reaches 95% with a < 5% major complication rate [65].

Recommendation

The initial imaging approach in patients with suspected PDA is TTE with Doppler. If the diagnosis cannot be confirmed, TEE is the next step. Cardiac MRI is seldom used or needed. Contrast angiography is utilized during percutaneous closure.

CHAPTER II

Left-Sided Obstructive Lesions

Wael AlJaroudi*[,1], Steve Lloyd[1], Ami E. Iskandrian[1] and Joel McLarry[2]

[1]*Division of Cardiovascular Disease, Department of Internal Medicine, University of Alabama at Birmingham, Birmingham, AL, USA*

[2]*Departments of Internal Medicine and Pediatrics, University of Alabama at Birmingham, Birmingham, AL, USA*

Abstract: Obstructive lesions impede the flow through the left-sided chambers and the left ventricular outflow. These lesions are cor triatriatum, congenital mitral stenosis, aortic coarctation, and subvalvular, valvular, and supravalvular aortic stenosis. In cor triatriatum and congenital mitral stenosis, echocardiography has a primary imaging role, with MRI and CC supplementing to help detect anomalous pulmonary veins and detect pressure gradients, respectively. TTE is the initial imaging for supravalvular and subvalvular aortic stenosis and MRI is utilized when TTE is non-diagnostic. Echocardiography plays a primary role in valvular aortic stenosis ,and MRI and CT are complementary for evaluating aortic aneurysms and coarctation. Because aortic coarctation is an extracardiac lesion, both MRI and CT can better visualize the defect and are therefore the primary imaging modalities.

1. COR TRIATRIATUM AND CONGENITAL MITRAL STENOSIS

Cor triatriatum consists of a common pulmonary venous chamber separated from the true left atrium inferiorly by a membrane. In severe cases, the membrane obstructs the blood flow, mimicking the physiology of mitral stenosis. It is usually an incidental finding, and is often associated with patent foramen ovale, ASD, persistent left superior vena cava, cleft mitral valve, or partial anomalous pulmonary venous drainage [66].

Congenital mitral stenosis is a rare entity with different forms: hypoplasia of the mitral valve annulus, commissural fusion, double orifice, thickened chordae tendinae, stenosing supravalvular ring and parachute mitral valve. It is commonly associated with coarctation of the aorta and aortic stenosis [2].

It is worth mentioning that multiple left sided obstructions can be present concomitantly in Shone's complex, including all or several of the following: supravalvular mitral ring, parachute mitral valve, subaortic stenosis, and aortic coarctation [67].

Role of Imaging

TTE with Doppler visualizes the membrane, estimates the gradient across the stenotic area, and screens for associated defects. A peak velocity >2 m/s indicates severe obstruction [39]. However, TTE lacks the ability to visualize the posterior rim of the membrane. TEE may confirm the diagnosis, though, in few reported cases, the orifice could only be visualized with transthoracic 3DE [68].

MRI is used to detect associated anomalous pulmonary veins, if clinically suspected (see Table **5**, p.13); CC measures the gradient across the membrane or stenotic valve, but cannot differentiate cor triatriatum from other left atrial inflow obstructive lesions [66]. CT and nuclear imaging have no defined roles for these lesions at present.

Recommendation

TTE is the preferred imaging modality. 3DE can complement the study to directly evaluate the orifice size thereby avoiding the pitfalls of Doppler. If anomalous pulmonary veins are suspected and not seen, TEE or MRI could prove useful.

*Corresponding Author: 701 19th Street, LHRB 306, Birmingham, AL 35294-0007, Alabama, USA; Tel: 205-934-0820; Fax: 205-934-7579; E-mail: wjaroudi@hotmail.com

Wael AlJaroudi (Ed.)

2. SUB-VALVULAR AORTIC STENOSIS

Sub-valvular aortic stenosis is due to a discrete fibrous membrane and/or muscular narrowing, which results in a focal obstruction (90% of cases), or a diffuse tunnel-like narrowing. It is associated with peri-membranous VSD in 37% of cases, and almost invariably with aortic regurgitation. Additionally, sub-valvular aortic stenosis can be acquired from interventricular septum misalignment during VSD closure [66].

Role of Imaging

M-mode echocardiography shows early closure and coarse fluttering of the aortic valve, a non-specific finding. 2DE parasternal long-axis view shows the subaortic membrane. The sensitivity of TTE improves in the apical long-axis or five chamber views. The role of 3DE has been described in few case reports [69].

TTE with Doppler shows a turbulent flow below the aortic valve. However, the pressure gradient may be underestimated if the LV function is depressed, or in the presence of a nonrestrictive VSD. A mean LV outflow gradient ≥50 mm Hg indicates severe stenosis that warrants surgery. Re-stenosis can occur in one third of surgically treated cases, and therefore, necessitates close monitoring for recurrence [66].

MRI provides useful information if echocardiography is non-diagnostic, aiding in clarifying anatomy and quantifying flow velocity [66]; CC is seldom necessary. Nuclear imaging and CT have no defined roles at present.

Recommendation

TTE with Doppler is the method of choice for diagnosis and follow-up for subvalvular aortic stensosis.

3. VALVULAR AORTIC STENOSIS

Almost 70% of the cases of valvular aortic stenosis consist of a bicuspid aortic valve which is also commonly associated with aortic root dilation and aortic regurgitation [66].

Role of Imaging

Long-axis parasternal TTE often shows doming of the aortic valve leaflets during systole; short-axis view confirms the diagnosis. The valve area is calculated using the continuity equation, or measured using valve planimetry by TEE or 3DE [21].

MRI and CT visualize the aortic valve leaflet and evaluate for thoracic aortic aneurysm and coarctation (Figure **3**). Unlike CT, MRI provides aortic valve velocity. Nuclear imaging has no role at the present and CC is seldom needed.

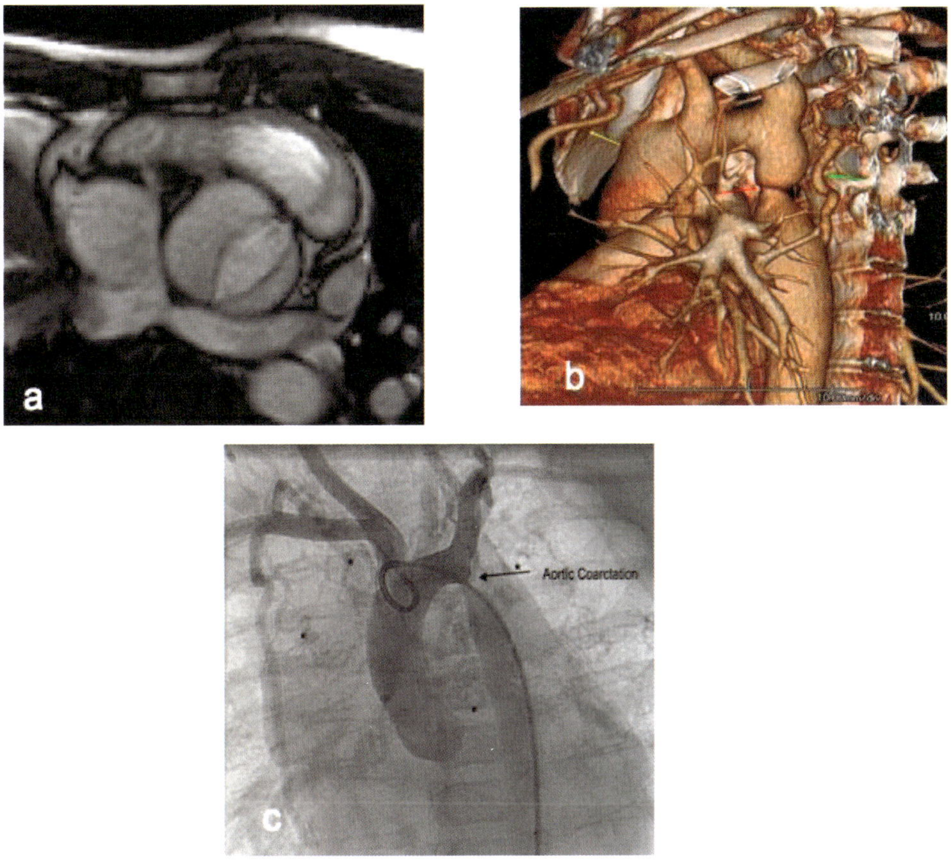

Figure 3. Bicuspid aortic valve and coarctation of aorta

(a) Cine-MRI of en face plane of the aortic valve showing bicuspid leaflets.

(b) CT angiogram with 3-dimensional reconstruction showing coarctation of the aorta (red arrow), dilated internal mammary artery (yellow artery), and dilated intercostal arteries (green arrow).

(c) Contrast angiogram depicting the coarctation of aorta (arrow) and multiple collateral vessels (asterix).

Recommendation

TTE is the imaging modality of choice for diagnosis and follow-up of valvular aortic stenosis.

4. SUPRA-VALVULAR AORTIC STENOSIS

It is defined by a narrowing at the sino-tubular junction that extends to the ascending aorta and can restrict coronary perfusion, potentially causing myocardial ischemia. It is often associated with Williams syndrome with concomitant mitral valve prolapse and pulmonary artery stenosis [66].

Role of Imaging

TTE with Doppler demonstrates the lesion and measures the gradient [39]; however, TEE is superior in evaluating the full extent of the ascending aorta [66].

MRI is used when echo is non-diagnostic [70]. Contrast angiography is seldom needed. Nuclear imaging may have a role if myocardial ischemia is suspected. CT has not been studied for this indication.

Recommendation

TTE with Doppler should be the initial imaging modality for the evaluation of aortic stenosis.

5. COARCTATION OF THE AORTA

Coarctation of the aorta consists of a discrete ridge that extends into the aortic lumen at the isthmus, distal to the left subclavian artery. It is associated with bicuspid aortic valve, VSD, PDA, mitral regurgitation, anomalous origin of the right subclavian artery, thoracic aortic aneurysm, and cerebral aneurysms. Potential complications include: HF, aortic dissection, premature coronary artery disease, and stroke. After repair, patients are at risk of re-coarctation or aneurysmal dilatation [71].

Role of Imaging

TTE is performed via the suprasternal view with continuous wave Doppler. This view might be suboptimal and can miss up to 50% of postoperative anomalies, such as re-coarctation, aortic arch hypoplasia, and pseudoaneurysm, especially in the presence of a PDA [72]. TTE also underestimates the length of the isthmus, and the vascular diameters [73]. Table 7 lists the advantages and limitations of different imaging modalities [66,74].

Table 7. Role of Imaging in Patients with Coarctation of the Aorta

Imaging Modality	Advantages	Disadvantages
2D TTE	Non invasive	Limited suprasternal view
	Widely available	↓ sensitivity in PDA present
	Assesses valvular/LV function	Arch, descending aorta not well seen
	Hemodynamic data	Collaterals not visualized
		Underestimate size of lesion
2D TEE	Available	Semi-invasive
	Descending thoracic aorta seen	Sedation
	Stent often visualized	Limited view of aortic arch
	Assesses valvular/LV function	Abdominal aorta not seen
	Ideal for intraoperative use	Collaterals not visualized
MRI	Non-invasive	Limited availability
	No radiation	Long procedure
	Non-iodine based contrast	Might require sedation
	Visualizes entire aortic tree	Underestimates isthmus size
	Visualizes collateral network	Artifact from stents
	3-dimensional images	Contraindications (pacemaker)
	High resolution in all planes	No intraoperative use
	Assesses valvular/LV function	
	Hemodynamic data	
	Ideal for follow up	
CT	Fast study	Radiation
	Non-invasive	Iodine contrast
	Visualizes the entire aortic tree	Limited availability
	Visualizes collateral network	Limited oblique view of arch
	3-dimensional images	Low resolution in sagittal plane
	Visualizes the stent	Calcium blooming artifact
		No hemodynamic data
		No intraoperative use
Angiography	Visualizes collateral network	Invasive
	Measures peak-peak gradient	Radiation
	Percutaneous repair	Iodine contrast
		Limited views (biplane)

Abbreviations: CT: computed tomography, LV: left ventricle, MRI: magnetic resonance imaging [Modified from references 66, 74].

In severe coarctation, a peak gradient ≥20 mm Hg is detected. TTE correlation with CC measurements is suboptimal [39], mainly due to variations in cardiac output, lesion length, aortic compliance and collaterals [75]. A high-grade antegrade flow that extends into diastole correlates with a hemodynamically significant lesion, but is less reliable in the presence of extensive collaterals [66]. TEE examines the entire thoracic aorta including prior stents, but with a limited view of the arch. TEE is ideal during repairs [74]. There are no published reports on the merits of 3DE.

MRI has a reported 100% sensitivity and specificity in detecting coarctation [76] and it can accurately measure the narrowest aortic lumen except at the isthmus [77]. The hemodynamic data correlate well with CC [78], but is underestimated when the imaging plane is misaligned with the flow, aliasing is present, or when temporal resolution is low [79,80]. Stent artifact is also a major limitation.

CT provides high resolution images (Figure **3b**) with short acquisition time and minimal stent artifact. Differences up to 9 mm in diameter size can be observed between MRI and CT, which introduces a significant source of error if different imaging modalities are used during the follow-up of a single patient [81].

The role of contrast angiography (Figure **3c**) is mostly limited to guidance of percutaneous interventions [82]. There is no defined role for nuclear imaging at present.

Recommendation

Cardiac MRI or CT is preferred for diagnosis but the same imaging modality should be used for follow-up. TEE is frequently used intraoperatively while contrast angiography is used during percutaneous interventions.

CHAPTER III

Cyanotic Heart Diseases

Wael AlJaroudi[*,1], Steve Lloyd[1], Ami E. Iskandrian[1] and Joel McLarry[2]

[1]*Division of Cardiovascular Disease, Department of Internal Medicine, University of Alabama at Birmingham, Birmingham, AL, USA*

[2]*Departments of Internal Medicine and Pediatrics, University of Alabama at Birmingham, Birmingham, AL, USA*

Abstract: Tetralogy of Fallot, Transposition of the Great Arteries, and the Fontan circulation comprise some of the most common congenital cyanotic lesions encountered in practice. Tetralogy can be repaired initially, if the lesion is severe enough, with a systemic-to-pulmonary shunt to augment pulmonary blood flow. Then the definitive repair closes the VSD and enlarges the RV outflow tract. TTE is the initial imaging study of choice for Tetralogy, however, MRI and sometimes CT complement to assess conduits and post-op pulmonary valve insufficiency. d-TGA is characterized by ventriculoarterial discordance and initially was repaired by an atrial switch and is now repaired by an arterial switch. CCTGA has atrioventricular in addition to ventriculoarterial discordance and therefore does not usually necessitate surgical repair. Initial imaging is done with TTE, but TEE, MRI, and CT are frequently required to image the baffle from an atrial switch repair. Contrast angiography is used during percutaneous intervention to repair baffle stenosis. The Fontan circulation is the result of a series of surgeries to repair single ventricle anatomies. TTE is the initial imaging modality, but MRI is usually needed to visualize the entire Fontan circuit. CT and TEE are sometimes used as alternatives.

1. TETRALOGY OF FALLOT

Tetralogy of Fallot is characterized by a VSD, overriding aorta, RV outflow tract obstruction, and RV hypertrophy (Figure **4**). Associated anomalies include: right–sided aortic arch (25%), ASD (10%), anomalous origin of coronary arteries (10%), and in most cases a dilated aortic root. Adult patients may present several years after repair with HF, pulmonary insufficiency, atrial arrhythmias or even sudden cardiac death [83].

Palliative shunts and corrective surgical procedures to increase pulmonary blood flow in Tetralogy of Fallot include (1) the Blalock-Taussig shunt (end-to-side anastomosis of the subclavian artery to the pulmonary artery) and the modified Blalock-Taussig shunt (Gore-Tex graft from the subclavian artery to pulmonary artery); (2) the Waterston shunt (side-to-side anastomosis of the ascending aorta to the right pulmonary artery); (3) the Potts shunt (side-to-side anastomosis of the descending aorta to the left pulmonary artery) (Figure 4e). The Waterston and Potts shunts are no longer used because of associated PHT and pulmonary artery deformation [83].

Corrective surgery requires patch closure of the VSD and enlargement of the RV outflow tract, which often renders the pulmonary valve incompetent. Patients may have an anomalous left anterior descending coronary artery arising from the right coronary artery coursing in front of the RV outflow tract, which can be severed during ventriculotomy [83].

Role of Imaging

The parasternal short-axis, subcostal coronal and sagittal views of TTE evaluate the RV outflow tract and pulmonary valve accurately. They demonstrate anterior deviation of the conal septum, and the infundibular muscle bundles. High velocity Doppler signal in the RV outflow tract indicates obstruction; however, there might be multiple obstructive lesions, and the most distal ones might be missed by TTE. The suprasternal view can be used to evaluate the aortic arch to rule out aortic root dilatation, which is being increasingly recognized as a risk factor for aortic dissection in this patient cohort [84]. However, the timing of surgical repair for aortic root dilatation remains controversial [39]. TTE with Doppler often misses pulmonary artery stenosis, especially if it involves the peripheral branches. Furthermore, it

*Corresponding Author: 701 19th Street, LHRB 306, Birmingham, AL 35294-0007, Alabama, USA; Tel: 205-934-0820; Fax: 205-934-7579; E-mail: wjaroudi@hotmail.com

Wael AlJaroudi (Ed.)

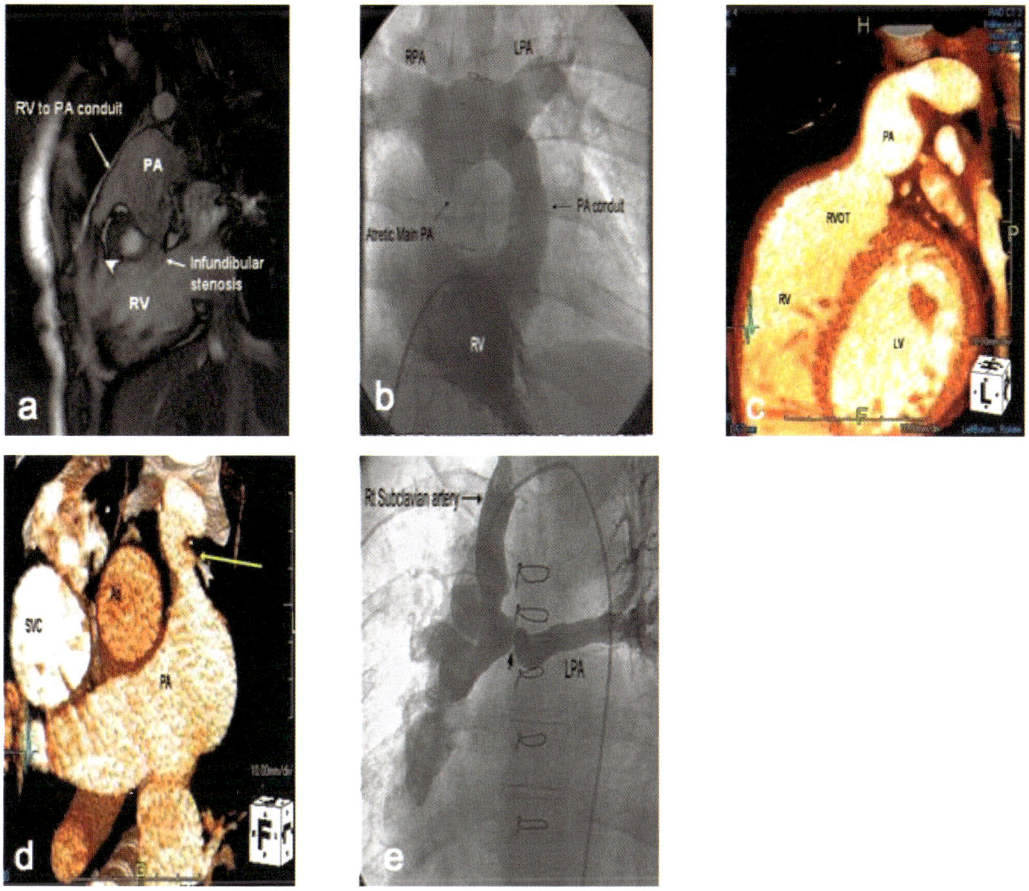

Figure 4. Tetralogy of Fallot

(a) Cine-MRI shows dilated RV with infundibular stenosis, and an RV to PA conduit with severe regurgitation (arrow head).

(b) Right ventriculogram shows flow from RV through a conduit into the LPA. The main pulmonary artery is atretic.

(c) Cardiac CT shows dilated RV outflow tract

(d) Cardiac CT shows infundibular stenosis (yellow arrow)

(e) Contrast angiogram shows a Blalock-Taussig shunt with a proximal stenosis in the LPA (arrow).

Abbreviations: Ao: aorta, LPA: left pulmonary artery, LV: left ventricle, PA: pulmonary artery, RPA: right pulmonary artery, RV: right ventricle, RVOT: right ventricular outflow tract, SVC: superior vena cava)

underestimates the trans-conduit gradient. TEE has similar limitations [39]. At present, the role of 3DE is not established.

MRI has superior spatial resolution, larger field of view, provides greater morphological information including peripheral pulmonary arteries, conduits, and anomalous origin of coronary arteries [85]. It is superior to TTE in determining RV hypertrophy and overriding aorta, and superior to contrast angiography in evaluating shunts, conduits, and pulmonary arteries. It identifies Blalock-Taussig shunts in 100% of cases [85], the proximal portion of the RV-pulmonary artery conduit in 93% of cases and its mid-portion in 100% of cases [86]. Additionally, MRI can be used to assess pulmonary regurgitation and RV volume, as it can be used to determine timing of pulmonary valve replacement for pulmonary insufficiency after initial tetralogy of Fallot repair (87). CT also performs well, producing high temporal and spatial resolution images (88). At the present, contrast angiography is limited to percutaneous pulmonary valvuloplasty and pulmonary artery dilatation. There is no defined role for nuclear imaging.

Recommendation

The evaluation should start with TTE, and be complemented with MRI or CT to assess the pulmonary arteries and conduits if necessary.

2. TRANSPOSITION OF THE GREAT ARTERIES

d-TGA is characterized by ventriculoarterial discordance (Figure **5**). Congenitally corrected transposition (CCTGA or l-TGA) has atrioventricular and ventriculoarterial discordance and, therefore, does not necessitate early surgical repair. CCTGA and post-operative d-TGA adults can present with multiple complications (Table **8**) [89].

Table 8. Clinical Findings in Adult Patients with Repaired Transposition of the Great Arteries

TGA	Surgery	Clinical issues	Clinical pearls
d-TGA	Atrial switch	Atrial flutter	14% of patients, marker of SCD
		Sinus node dysfunction	11% will need a pacemaker
		RV dysfunction	Unknown benefit of HF medications
		Tricuspid regurgitation	Due to annular dilation
		Anomalous coronary arteries	LCx from RCA (22%), Single RCA (9.5%), Single left coronary (3%), inverted coronaries (3%)
		Baffle stenosis	SVC obstruction is the most common
			Dilation prior to lead implantation
			PHT if on pulmonary venous side
		Baffle leak	More common than stenosis
			Risk for paradoxical embolization
		PHT	7% of adults
	Arterial switch	Coronary artery stenosis	Might cause SCD
		Distorted pulmonary artery	Stenosis at anastomosis site
		Dilated aortic root	Common finding
		Aortic insufficiency	Due to aortic root dilation
CCTGA	None	RV dysfunction	Due to tricuspid regurgitation
		Arrhythmias	High morbidity
		Tricuspid regurgitation	Needs valve replacement
		Complete heart block	2% incidence/year
		Pulmonary stenosis	40% of patients
		VSD	70% of patients, perimembranous

Abbreviations: HF: heart failure, LCx: left circumflex coronary artery, PHT: pulmonary hypertension, RCA: right coronary artery, RV: right ventricle, SCD: sudden cardiac death, SVC: superior vena cava, VSD: ventricular septal defect, CCTGA: congenitally corrected TGA. [Modified from reference 89].

The Senning procedure or atrial switch was the first corrective procedure for d-TGA, first performed in 1958 by creating a baffle from autologous tissue that directed the systemic venous return to the pulmonary artery, and the pulmonary venous return into the aorta. The Mustard procedure is a similar operation but the baffle is created from a synthetic material [89]. Both the Senning and Mustard procedures utilize the RV as the systemic chamber, and therefore systemic RV failure is a major complication in these patients as they progress into adulthood. The currently preferred operation for d-TGA, the arterial switch, was first performed in 1976; the great arteries are transected and switched into their new positions, and the coronary arteries are detached with a button of tissue and sutured in the new aorta [89].

Role of Imaging

A long-axis TTE view shows an enlarged morphological RV (systemic ventricle) with a posteriorly pushed ventricular septum into a small banana-shaped LV, which often causes LV outflow tract obstruction. Common findings include: systolic anterior movement of the mitral valve leaflet, fluttering and premature closure of the pulmonary valve, and dynamic turbulent flow in the LV outflow tract [39]. TTE is often limited by poor acoustic window. TEE is more sensitive in detecting all types of baffle leaks and obstructions. The longitudinal plane visualizes the inferior limb, while the transverse plane visualizes the superior limb, pulmonary venous atrium, and baffle leaks. 3-DE can visualize an intraatrial baffle obstruction in long-axis and in en-face view [90]. The Doppler signal in the baffle is usually triphasic but loses its pulsatility in the presence of obstruction [39]. TTE correctly identifies pulmonary artery anastomosis stenosis, a common complication after arterial switch, but evaluates peripheral branch pulmonary artery stenosis with difficulty [39].

MRI visualizes the intraatrial baffle in multiple planes and detects all types of malfunction [91, 92]. 3D-MRA allows accurate evaluation of peripheral pulmonary artery branch stenosis and anastomosis narrowing. Time resolved 3D-MRA can also detect pulmonary hypertension and accurately calculate mean pulmonary arterial pressure [93].

CT provides similar information to MRI. Contrast angiography is used for percutaneous balloon dilatation and stenting of systemic baffle stenosis (see Table **6**, p.17). There is no defined role for nuclear imaging at present.

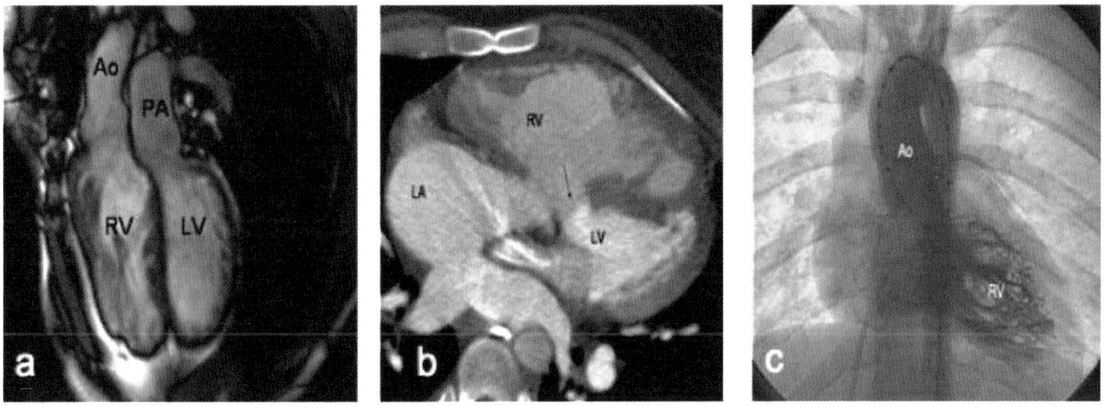

Figure 5. Transposition of the Great Arteries (TGA)

a. Cine MRI view shows ventricularterial discordance in a patient with d-TGA.

b. CT of a patient with d-TGA and a communicating VSD (arrow).

c. Contrast ventriculography showing the RV connected to the aorta.

Abbreviations: Ao: aorta, LA: left atrium, LV: left ventricle, PA: pulmonary artery, RV: right ventricle,), VSD: ventricular septal defect).

Recommendation

In TGA, TEE, MRI or CT are used to rule out baffle leak, stenosis or obstruction. Contrast angiography is used during stenting of superior vena cava-baffle narrowing.

3. THE FONTAN CIRCULATION

Adults survive tricuspid atresia, hypoplastic left heart syndrome, and other single ventricle configurations as a result of a series of palliative and reparative operations [94]. The Fontan operation is the final procedure in this series and it diverts the total caval blood flow directly to the pulmonary arteries. Potential long-term complications include arrhythmia, HF, conduit stenosis and thrombus formation (9%-11% incidence of thrombus in Fontan patients with 18% associated mortality) [95, 96].

Role of Imaging

The Fontan circuit might be too posterior to be appropriately imaged by TTE [92]. It is difficult to view areas of stenosis even with Doppler because of normal low flow velocity [39]. In addition, TTE often misses intra-conduit thrombus.

TEE, on the other hand, is particularly useful in detecting thrombus [97], residual shunt, and the posterior anastomoses [39]. The role of 3DE in evaluating the Fontan circuit has not been studied.

MRI clearly visualizes the Fontan circuit. Time resolved 3D-MRA assesses the flow dynamics in the Fontan circuit, which could only be visualized by contrast angiography [97]. In addition, it accurately detects thrombus [98,99]. CT can be used as an alternative test. The diagnostic role of contrast angiography has diminished with the increasing use of non-invasive alternatives. There is no known role for nuclear imaging.

Recommendation

Despite its limitations in Fontan patients, TTE is the initial evaluation, assessing ventricular and valvular function. MRI is the preferred imaging modality to evaluate the entire Fontan circulation and the complex morphology in repaired single ventricle physiology. CT or TEE could be used as alternatives.

CHAPTER IV

Other Congenital Cardiac Lesions

Wael AlJaroudi*[,1], Steve Lloyd[1], Ami E. Iskandrian[1] and Joel McLarry[2]

[1]*Division of Cardiovascular Disease, Department of Internal Medicine, University of Alabama at Birmingham, Birmingham, AL, USA*

[2]*Departments of Internal Medicine and Pediatrics, University of Alabama at Birmingham, Birmingham, AL, USA*

Abstract: Ebstein's anomaly is an abnormality of the tricuspid valve in which there is a failure of delamination, resulting in tethering of septal and posterior leaflets, apical displacement of the functional annulus and atrialization of the RV. TTE complemented by 3DE is used to diagnose and evaluate for surgical repair. Several congenital heart defects also concomitantly have anomalous origin of their coronary arteries. Some anomalous coronaries, such as an anomalous coronary arising from the opposite sinus, are associated with sudden cardiac death, making their detection imperative. TTE often fails to visualize the coronary arteries. TEE has increased sensitivity, but MRI and MR and CT angiography is the standard to detect anomalous coronaries and elucidate their course.

1. EBSTEIN'S ANOMALY

Ebstein's anomaly is an abnormality of the tricuspid valve in which there is failure of delamination, resulting in tethering of septal and posterior leaflets, apical displacement of the functional annulus and atrialization of the RV. The valve is invariably regurgitant with occasional stenosis. 80% of patients have ASD or patent foramen ovale [83].

Role of Imaging

M-mode echocardiography shows paradoxical septal motion, dilated right atrium, and delayed closure of the tricuspid valve leaflets >65 ms after the mitral valve closure. These findings however, are non-specific. TTE shows abnormal septal leaflet attachment, RA dilatation, and tricuspid regurgitation. The most specific sign is the apical displacement of the septal leaflet from the mitral valve annulus to an extent greater than 8 mm/m^2 body surface area. The absence of this sign and the presence of non-redundant anterior leaflet have a 100% negative predictive value [39]. The specificity of TTE decreases in conditions that mimic Ebstein's anomaly such as tricuspid valve dysplasia, traumatic rupture, prolapse, and RV dysplasia [100]. TTE is of limited value in delineating areas of non-tethering, which have important implications during surgical repair [101]. 3DE has the advantage of multi-plane imaging in assessing the degree of tethering, bubble sign, rotation of hinge points, and abnormalities of tension apparatus [101]. MRI is generally not indicated [70], but may have a role in patients with poor acoustic windows [102]. CT, nuclear and contrast angiography do not have defined roles at present.

Recommendation

TTE complemented with 3DE should be the first imaging modality for diagnosis and evaluation of the appropriateness for surgical repair.

2. ANOMALOUS ORIGIN OF CORONARY ARTERIES

Congenital anomalies of the coronary arteries affect 1% of the general population and 3%-36% of adults with CHD (see Figures **6** and **7** and Table **9**) [103, 104].

*Corresponding Author: 701 19th Street, LHRB 306, Birmingham, AL 35294-0007, Alabama, USA; Tel: 205-934-0820; Fax: 205-934-7579; E-mail: wjaroudi@hotmail.com

Wael AlJaroudi (Ed.)

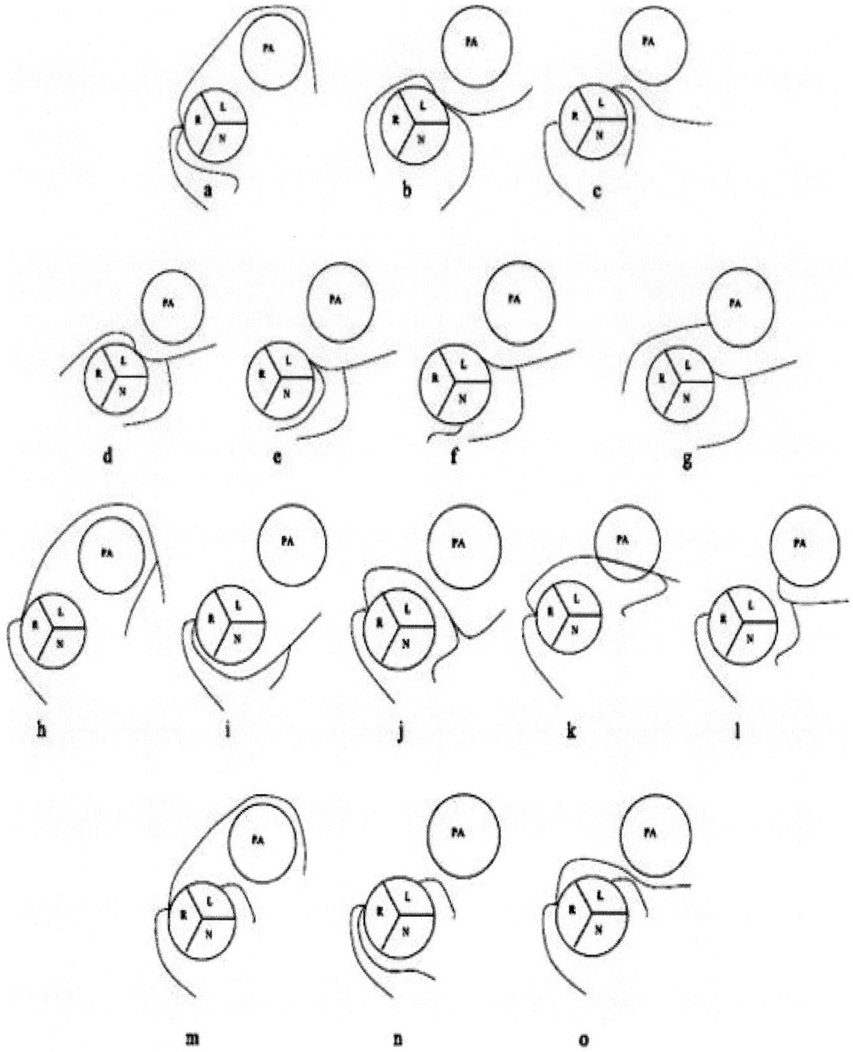

Figure 6. Schematic illustration of the origin and course of anomalous origin of coronary arteries.

(a) Separate origins from the right coronary sinus.

(b) Separate origins from the left coronary sinus.

(c) Separate ostium of the left circumflex coronary artery.

(d) Right coronary artery from the left coronary sinus with inter-arterial course.

(e) Right coronary artery from the left coronary sinus with retro-aortic course.

(f) Right coronary artery from the non coronary sinus.

(g) Right coronary artery from the pulmonary artery.

(h) Left main coronary artery from the right coronary sinus, anterior course.

(i) Left main coronary artery from the right coronary sinus, posterior course.

(j) Left man coronary artery from the right coronary sinus, inter-arterial course.

(k) Left main coronary artery from the right coronary sinus, subpulmonic course.

(l) Left main coronary artery from the pulmonary artery.

(m) Left anterior descending coronary artery from the right coronary sinus, anterior course.

(n) Left anterior descending coronary artery from the right coronary sinus, posterior course.

(o) Left anterior descending coronary artery from the right coronary sinus, inter-arterial course.

Abbreviations: L: left coronary cusp, N: non-coronary cusp, R: right coronary cusp.
[Modified from reference 107]

Table 9. Common Anomalous Coronary Arteries in Congenital Heart Disease

Tetralogy of Fallot	Enlarged conal artery
	LCA from RCA, anterior to RV outflow tract
	Single RCA
	Left circumflex to pulmonary artery
	RCA from left common coronary
	Anomalous left coronary artery from pulmonary artery
d-Transposition great arteries	RCA from posterior right sinus of Valsalva
	Left common artery from posterior left sinus of Valsalva
	Left circumflex artery from RCA
	Coronary artery inversion
	Intramural course
Congenitally corrected transposition great arteries	RCA from posterior aorta
	Left coronary from anterior aorta
Congenital mitral stenosis	Left coronary artery from RCA
Tricuspid atresia	Absent RCA
Bicuspid aortic valve	Anomalous left coronary artery from pulmonary artery
	Left coronary artery from RCA, anterior course
Coarctation of the aorta	Anomalous left coronary artery from pulmonary artery
Patent ductus arteriosus	Anomalous left coronary artery from pulmonary artery

Abbreviations: LCA: left common coronary artery, RCA: right coronary artery, RV: right ventricle. [Modified from reference 104].

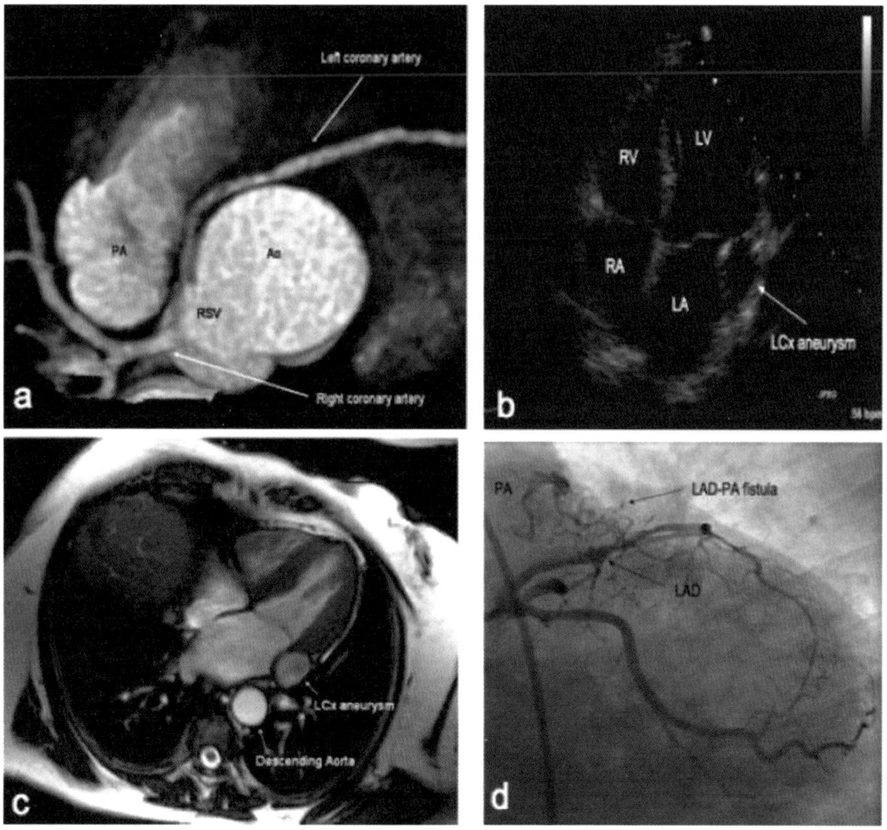

Figure 7. Anomalous origin of coronary arteries

(a) CT angiogram showing an anomalous left coronary artery from the right sinus of Valsalva with inter-arterial course. (ALCAPA).

(b) Four chamber TTE showing a left circumflex coronary artery aneurysm.

(c) Two chamber cine-MRI showing the left circumflex coronary artery aneurysm.

(d) Coronary angiogram showing a fistula between the left anterior descending coronary artery and the pulmonary artery.

Abbreviations: LA: left atrium, LAD: left anterior descending coronary artery, LCX: left circumflex coronary artery, LV: left ventricle, PA: pulmonary artery, RA: right atrium, RSV: right sinus of Valsalva, RV: right ventricle.

Role of Imaging

TTE has a relatively low sensitivity for the detection of coronary artery anomalies in adults and fails to show the origin of the coronary artery in many patients (Table **10**) [105-108]. Its role in identifying drainage sites of fistulas is also controversial [109]. Conversely, TEE frequently identifies the origin of the anomalous vessel (particularly left main) with up to 100% sensitivity [110]. At present, the role of 3DE is undefined although it has been examined in a single case report [111].

MRI and MR angiography are the current standard of care in the evaluation of anomalous coronaries [70]. MRI has a sensitivity and specificity of more than 95% in these conditions [101]. It detects the origin, course, morphology, and presence of plaques, thrombus, and ischemia (Table **10**). However, MRI has lower spatial resolution than cardiac CT [112], and is limited in the presence of arrhythmias, fast heart rates (>85), and metal artifacts.

64 slice detector CT is more sensitive than contrast angiography, and has a higher spatial resolution than MR angiography [107, 108]. However, the image quality is affected by vessel calcifications and arrhythmias. Furthermore, radiation exposure can be significant with CT especially in young patients.

The angiographic features of the different forms of these anomalies and their course were well described by Ishikawa et al in 1985 [113]. Coronary intravascular ultrasound (IVUS) can help identify the aortic intramural course of an anomalous vessel, which is associated with an interarterial course between the great arteries and sudden cardiac death [114]. Nuclear imaging might be used to detect myocardial ischemia in select patients [115, 116].

Table 10. Comparison of Imaging Techniques for Anomalous Coronary Arteries

	TTE	TEE	MRA	CTA	SCA	IVUS
Spatial resolution (mm)	0.8 x 1.5	0.8 x 1.0	0.7x0.7x1.5	0.5x0.5x0.5	0.3 x 0.3	0.15x 0.25
Temporal resolution (ms)	30	30	70	85	15	Variable
X-ray source	None	None	None	+++	++	None
Breath hold (s)	None	None	None	15-20	None	None
Contrast	None	None	Gadolinium	Iodine	Iodine	None
Visualizes origin of artery	+	+++	+++	+++	+++	+++
Visualizes course of artery	None	+	+++	+++	++	+
Evaluates intramural course	None	None	None	None	None	+++
Assess surrounding structures	++	+++	+++	+++	None	Limited
Characterizes tissue	+	+	+++	++	None	++
Dimensional views	2	2	3	3	2	2
Evaluates fistulas	+	++	++	+++	+++	None
Study duration (min)	15	30	20-60	15	30	45
Limitations	↓ sensitivity	Semi-invasive	Metal artifact, Arrhythmias	Calcification, Arrhythmias	Invasive	Invasive

Abbreviations: CTA: computed tomographic angiography, IVUS: intravascular ultrasound, MRA: magnetic resonance angiography, SCA: selective coronary angiography, TEE: transesophageal echocardiography, TTE: transthoracic echocardiography. [Modified from references 105-108]

Recommendation

When evaluating anomalous coronary arteries, TTE has a limited role, whereas MRI and CT are useful in the diagnosis of the anomalous origin of coronary arteries and elucidating their course.

Imaging Risks

Many of the imaging modalities discussed above can have damaging side effects when evaluating adults with congenital heart disease. Though there are no known serious risks from ultrasound, CT and MRI can pose serious risks. The associated radiation exposure from CT increases risk of malignancy by a small percentage with each scan, potentially creating significant risk in the congenital heart disease patient that requires multiple CTs over a lifetime [117]. Additionally, iodinated contrast carries risk as well, including acute kidney injury and allergic reactions. Outside of the presence of metal implants, MRI has no known serious risks by itself; however, gadolinium contrast has been associated with nephrogenic systemic fibrosis in renal failure patients in a dose dependent manner. Nephrogenic systemic fibrosis involves fibrosis of skin, joints, eyes, and internal organs and mainly occurs in end-stage renal patients on dialysis [118]. Less commonly it occurs in acute kidney injury and renal transplant patients. Contrast angiography carries the same risks of iodinated contrast and radiation exposure as CT, but typically the risk is increased by larger amounts of contrast and for prolonged procedures large doses of radiation as well.

CONCLUSIONS

In conclusion, each imaging modality has advantages and limitations in diagnosis and follow-up of adults with CHD and these imaging methods should complement thorough clinical evaluation and standard tests such as electrocardiography and chest radiography as a part of coordinated care by experienced adult congenital heart disease teams [58].

ACKNOWLEDGEMENTS

We thank Ray J Kim, MD, from the Duke Cardiovascular Magnetic Resonance Center, Durham, NC for providing us with Figures **2b**, **2c**, **2e**, **3a**, **4a**, **5a**, **7b**, **7c**, **24-31**, and **33**; William McMahon, MD, from the Department of Pediatric Cardiology, University of Alabama at Birmingham, Birmingham, AL, for providing us with Figures **3c**, **4b**, **4e**, **5c**, **16-21**, and **32**; Vijay Misra, MD, Department of Cardiovascular disease, University of Alabama at Birmingham, Birmingham, AL, for providing us with Figures **2a** and **7d**; Michael Ridner, MD, Department of Cardiovascular Disease, The Heart Center, Huntsville, AL, for providing us with Figure **7a**; Satinder Singh, MD, from the Department of Radiology, University of Alabama at Birmingham, Birmingham, AL, for providing us with Figures **3b**, **4c**, **4d**, **5b**, **22**, and **23**.

Appendix A: Cardiac Images of Congenital Heart Disease

ABBREVİATİONS

2DE: Two- Dimensional Echocardiography

3DE: Three-Dimensional Echocardiography

AS: Aortic Stenosis

ASD: Atrial Septal Defect

AV: Aortic Valve

CCTGA: Congenitally Corrected Transposition of the Great Arteries

CT: Computed Tomography

D-TGA: Dextro Transposition of the Great Arteries

LV: Left Ventricle/Ventricular

MRA: Magnetic Resonance Angiography

MRI: Magnetic Resonance Imaging

PA: Pulmonary Artery

PDA: Patent Ductus Arteriosus

PS: Pulmonic Stenosis

RV: Right Ventricle/Ventricular

TEE: Transesophageal Echocardiography

TGA: Transposition of the Great Arteries

TTE: Transthoracic Echocardiography

VSD: Ventricular Septal Defect

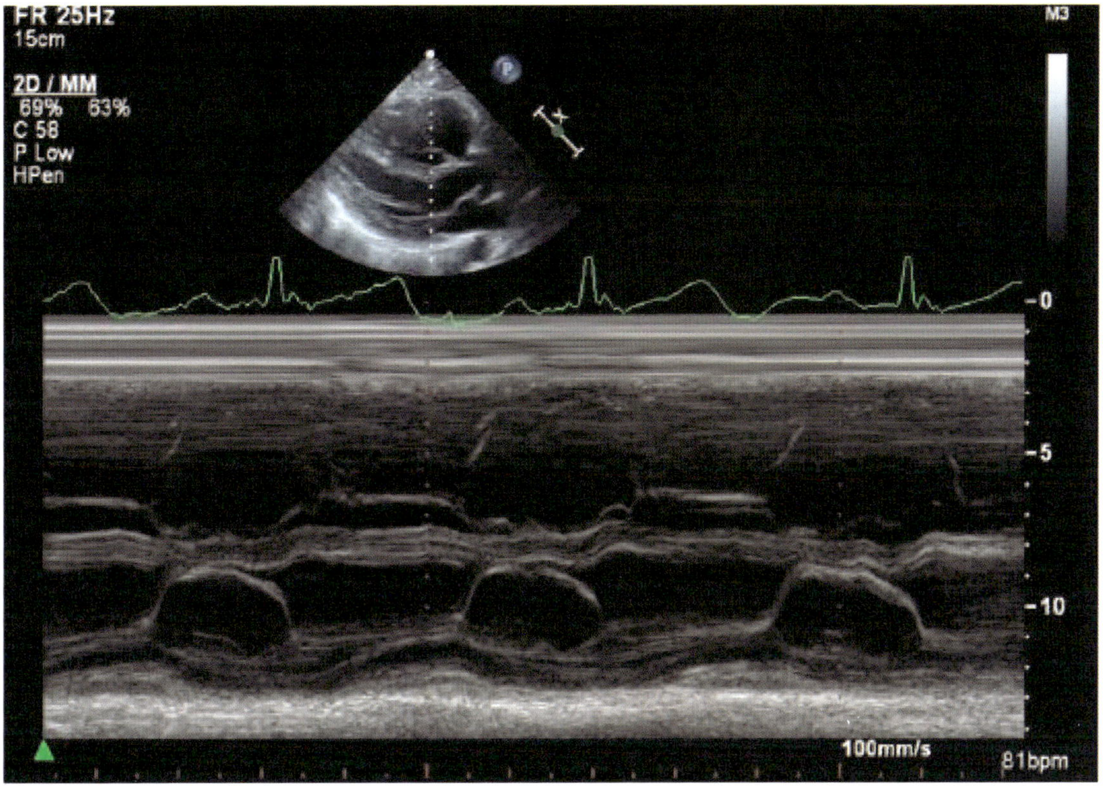

Figure 8a. 2D Echo M-mode of Ebstein's Anomaly Illustrating a Redundant Tricuspid Valve Leaflet.

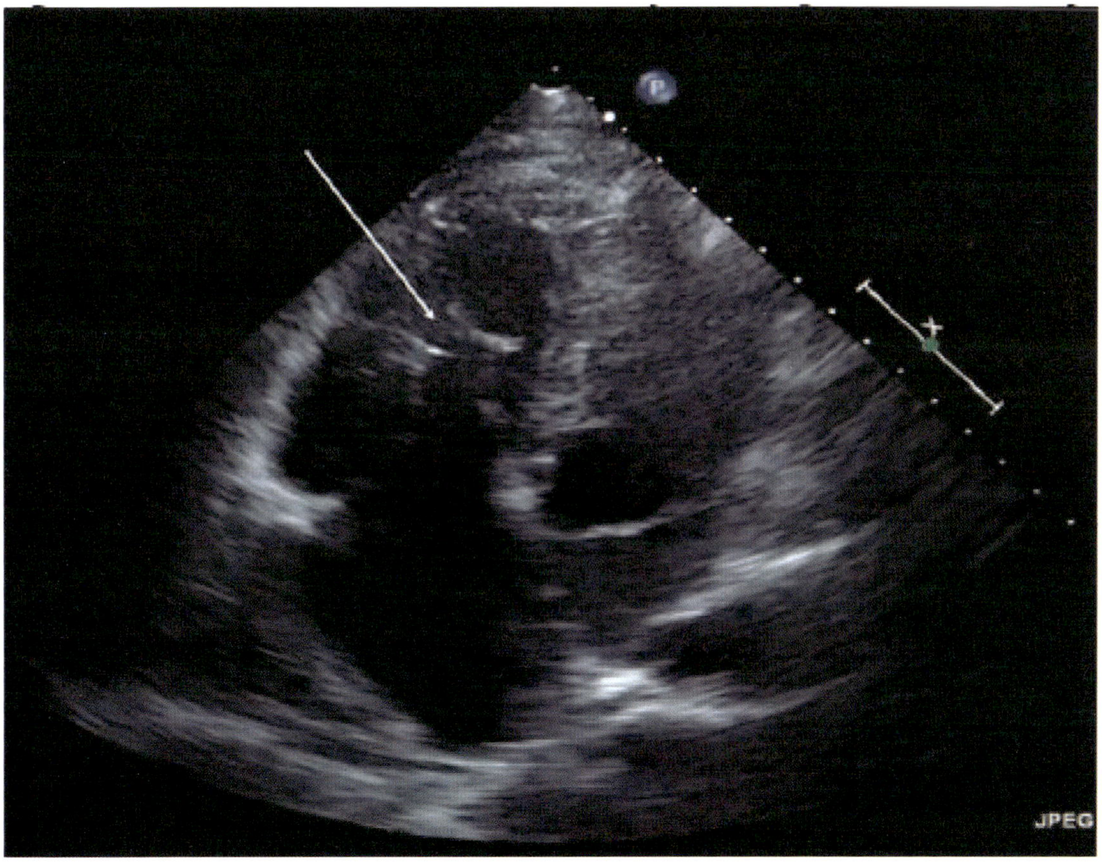

Figure 8b. 2D Echo showing failure of delamination of the tricuspid septal leaflet and atrialization of the right ventricle.

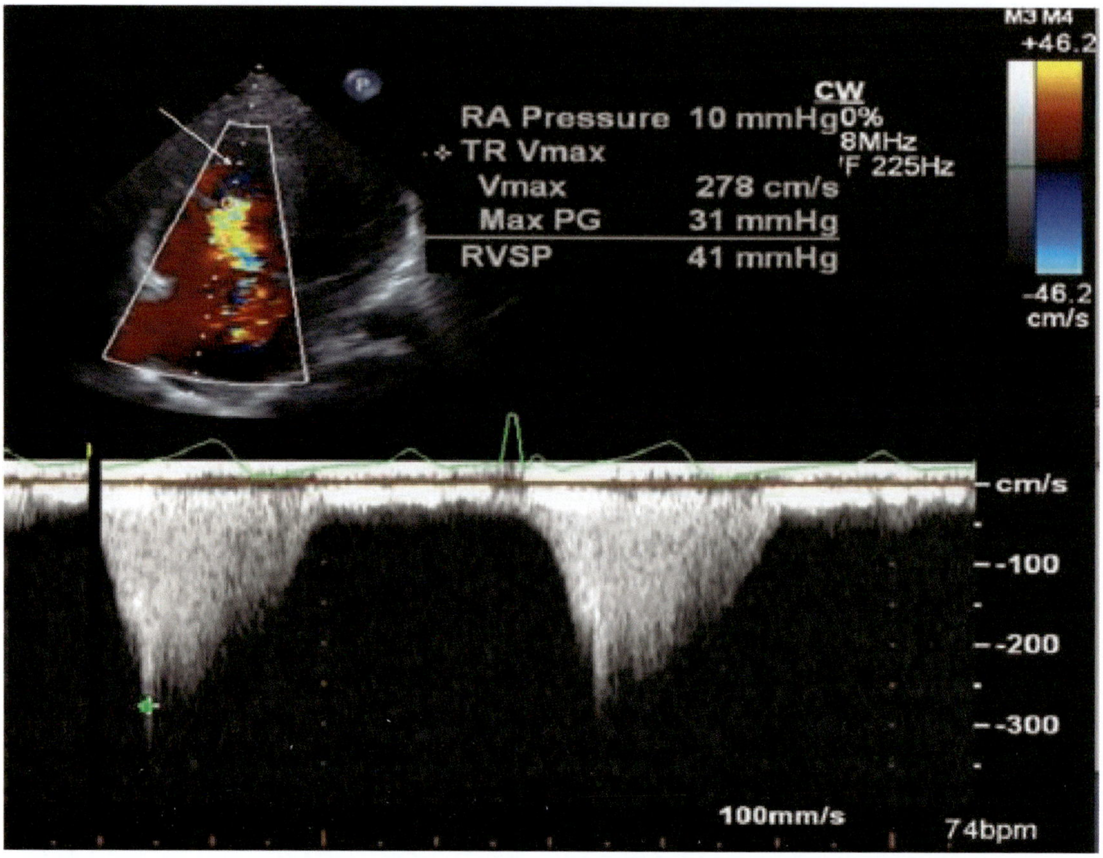

Figure 8c. 2D Echo with color Doppler showing tricuspid regurgitation originating near the apex.

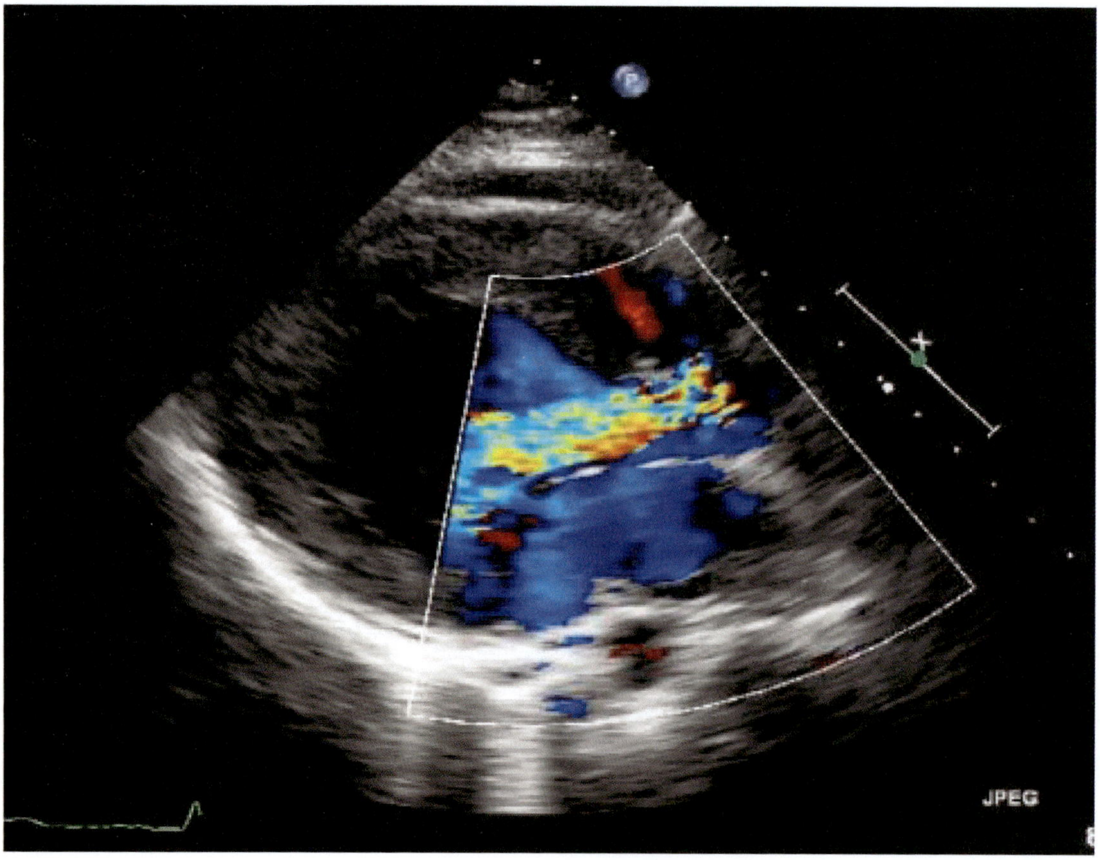

Figure 9a. 2D Echo with color of a patient with bicuspid aortic valve showing severe aortic insufficiency.

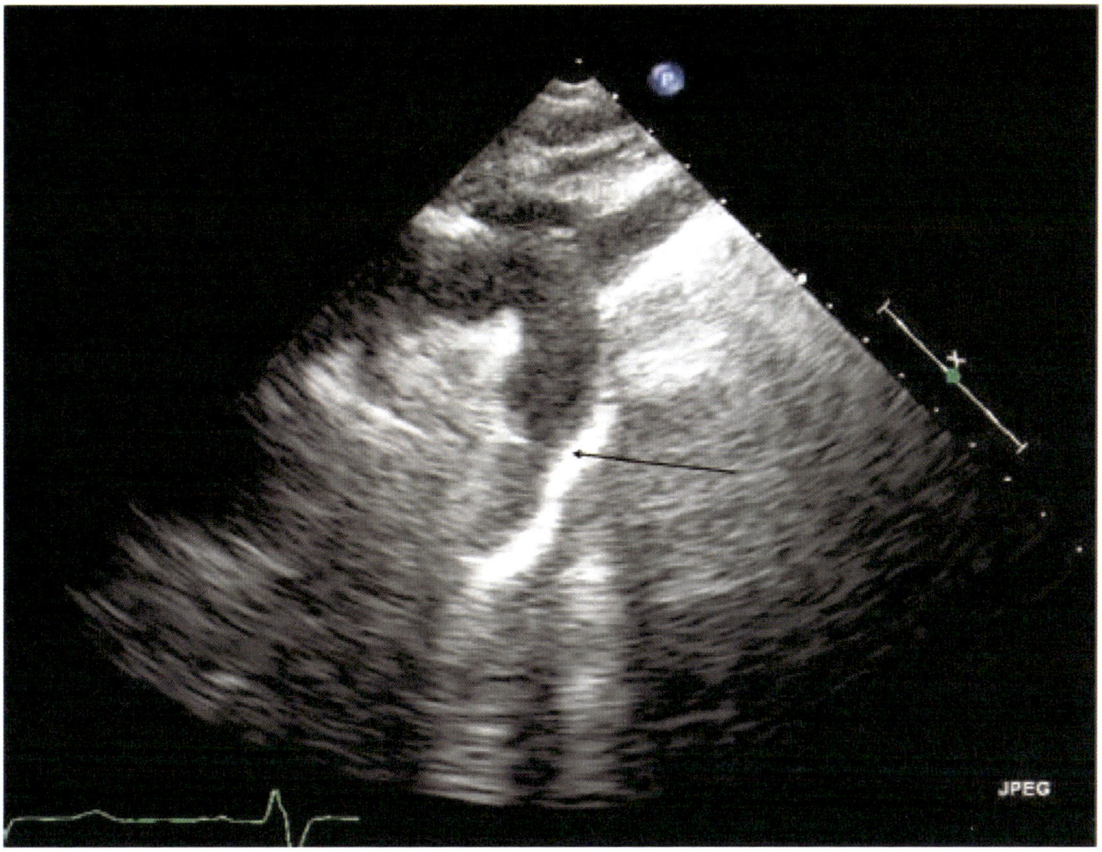

Figure 9b. Suprastenal view (2D echo) showing aortic coarctation (black arrow).

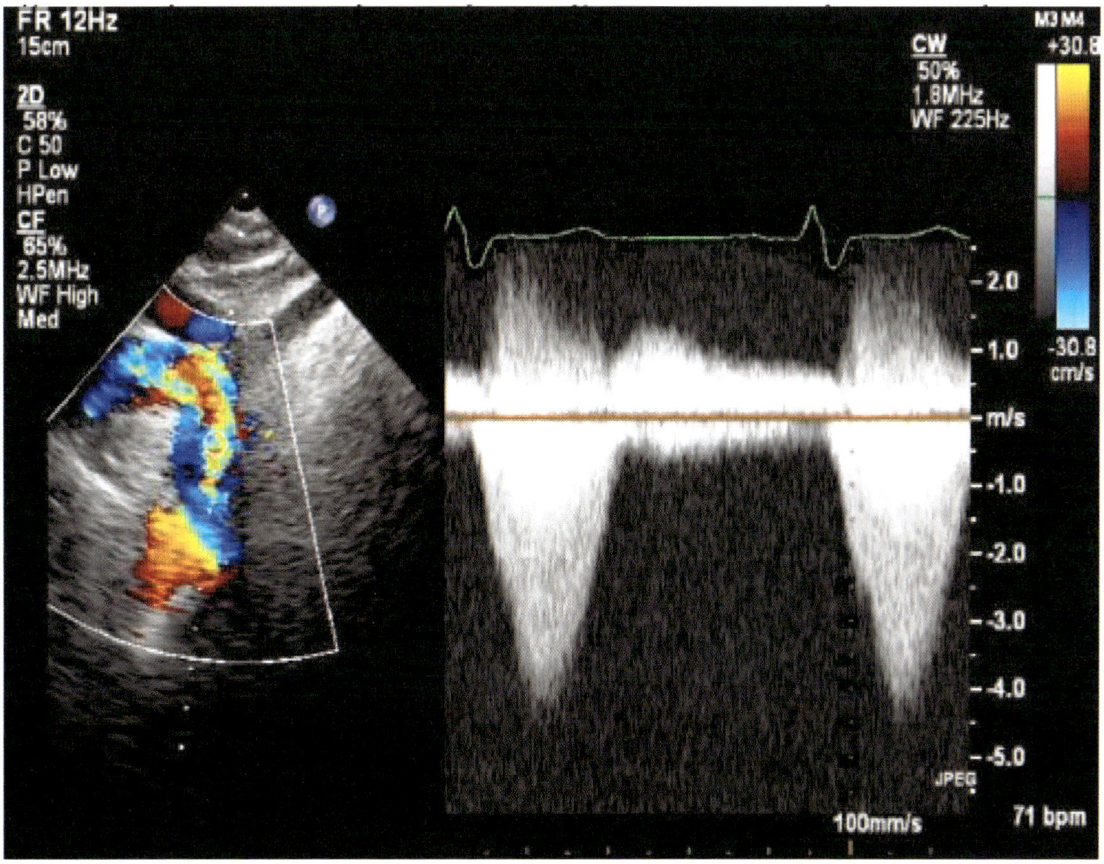

Figure 9c. 2D echo with color showing turbulent flow at the site of coarctation indicating significant stenosis.

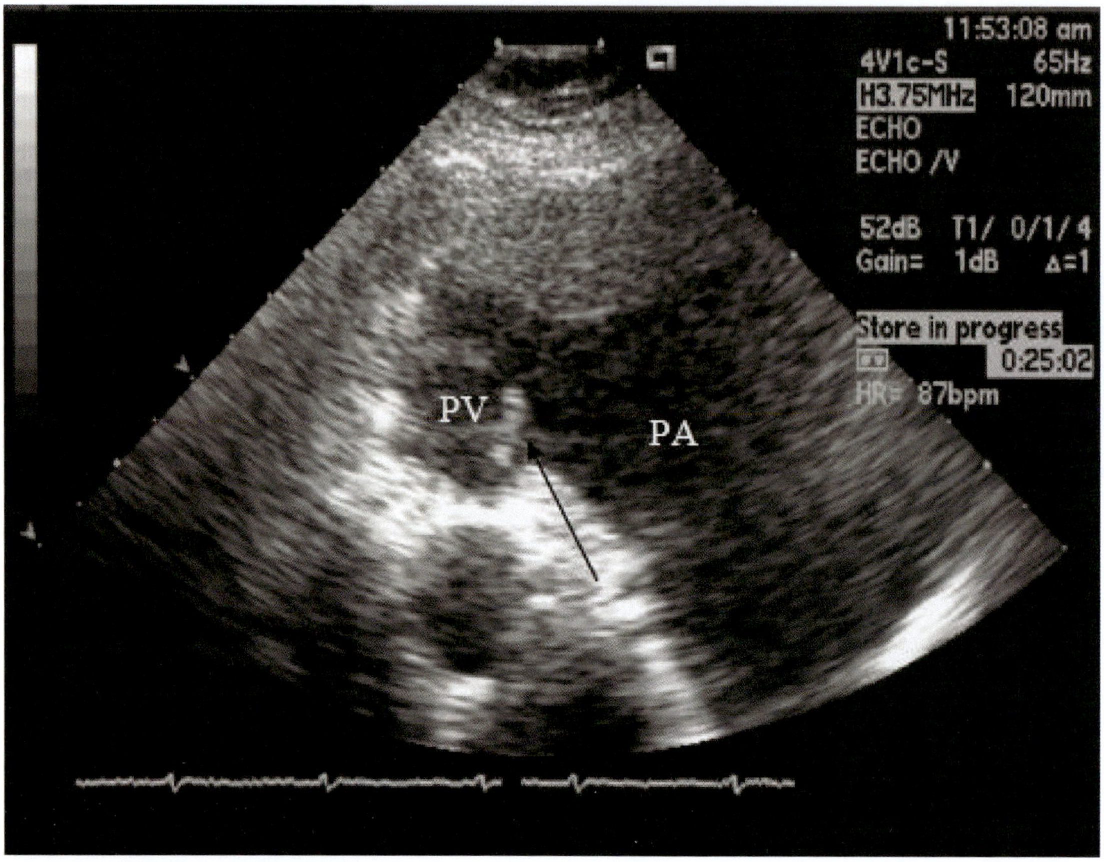

Figure 10. 2D Echo. Pulmonic Stenosis with Dilated Pulmonary Artery.

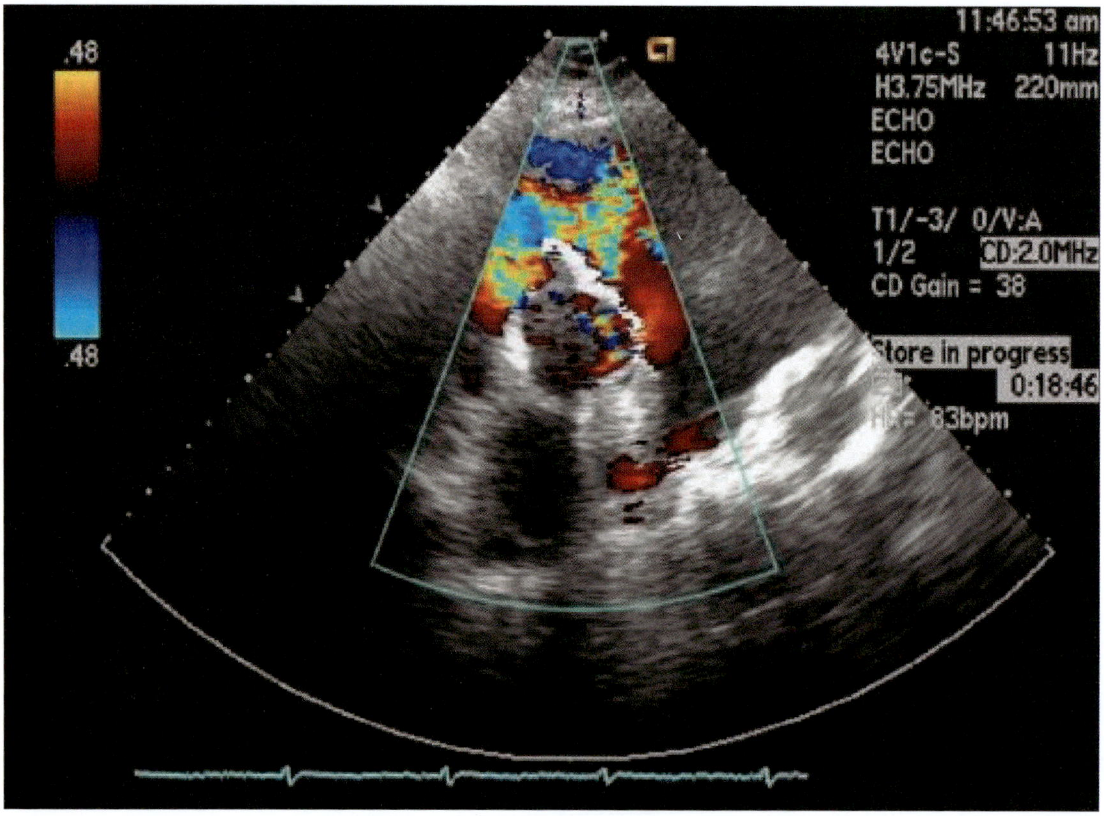

Figure 11. Pulmonic Stenosis with a pressure gradient and turbulent flow.

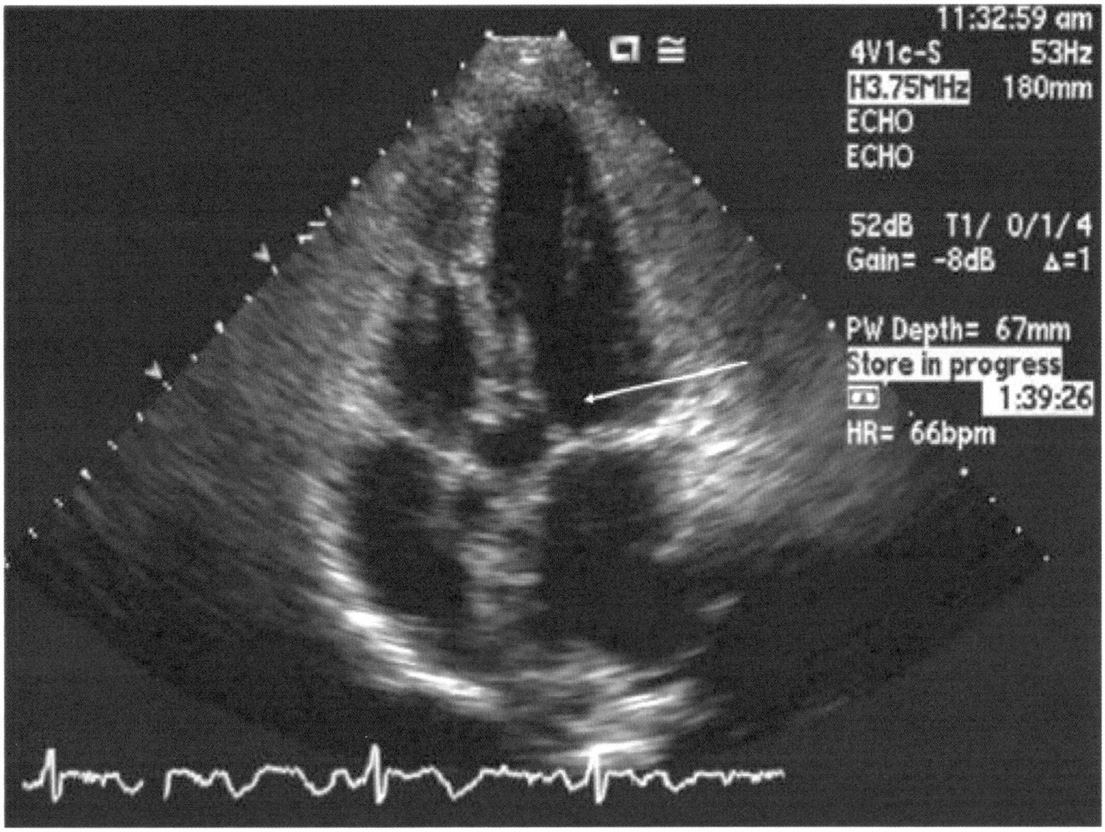

Figure 12. 2D Echo, five apical chamber view showing discrete subaortic membrane (arrow).

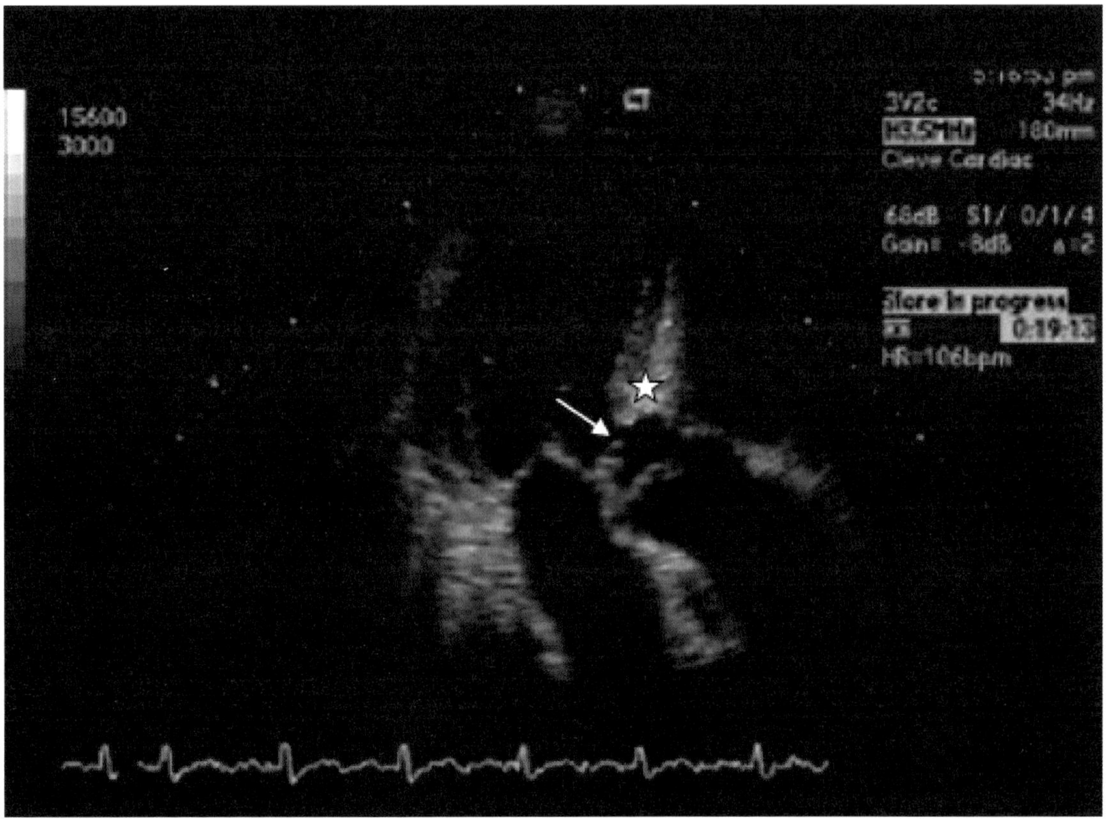

Figure 13. 2D echo, 3 chamber apical view showing subaortic membrane (arrow) and a vegetation (star).

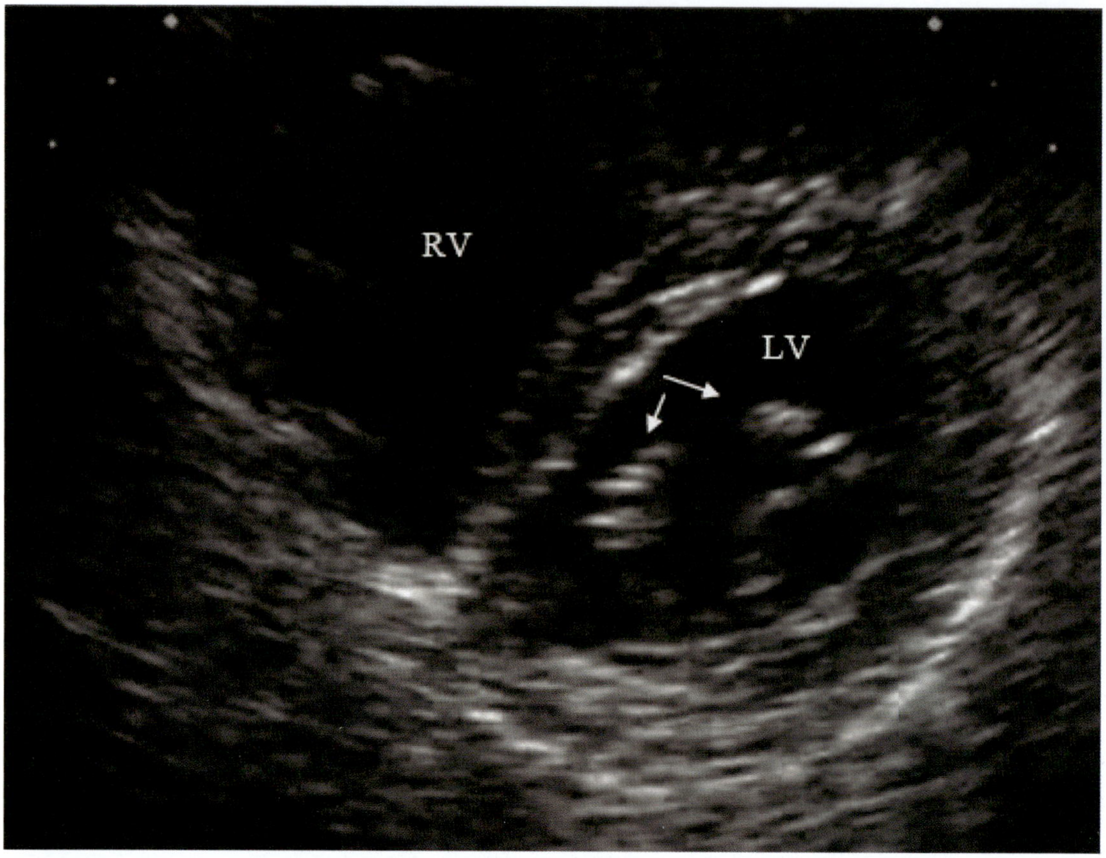

Figure 14. 2D Echo. Primum ASD with cleft mitral valve (arrows).

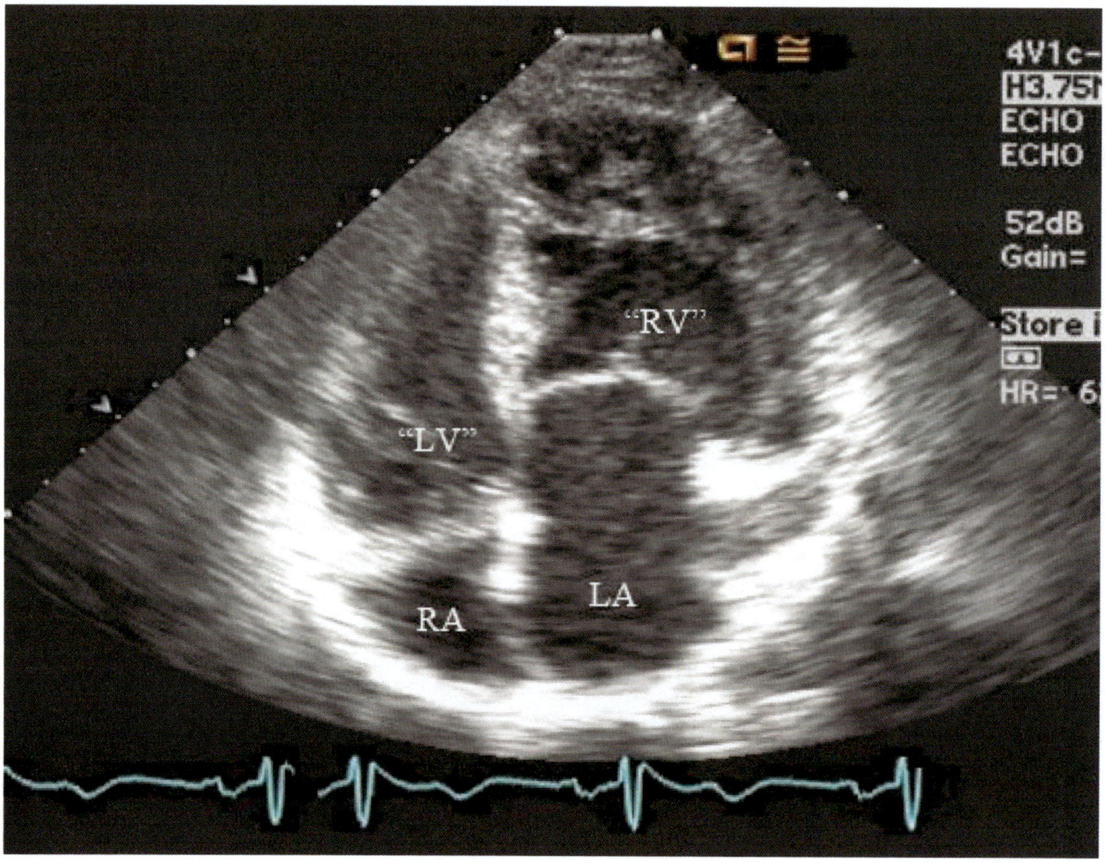

Figure 15. CCTGA with morphologic but also systemic right ventricle.

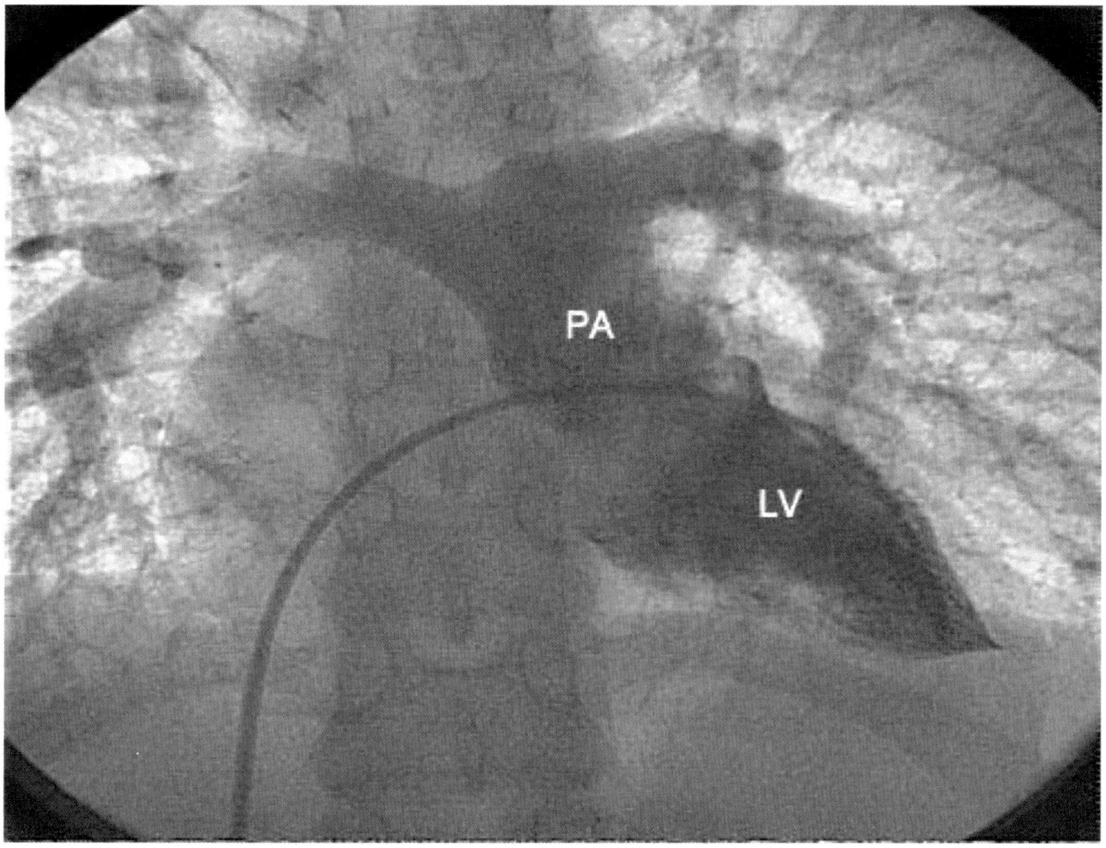

Figure 16. Arteriogram of D-TGA showing LV to PA connection.

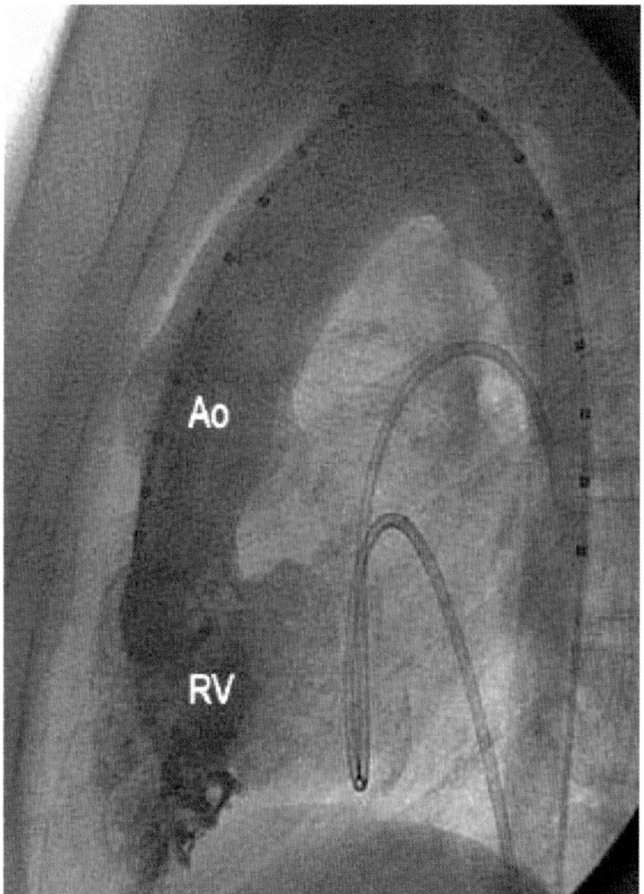

Figure 17. Arteriogram of D-TGA.

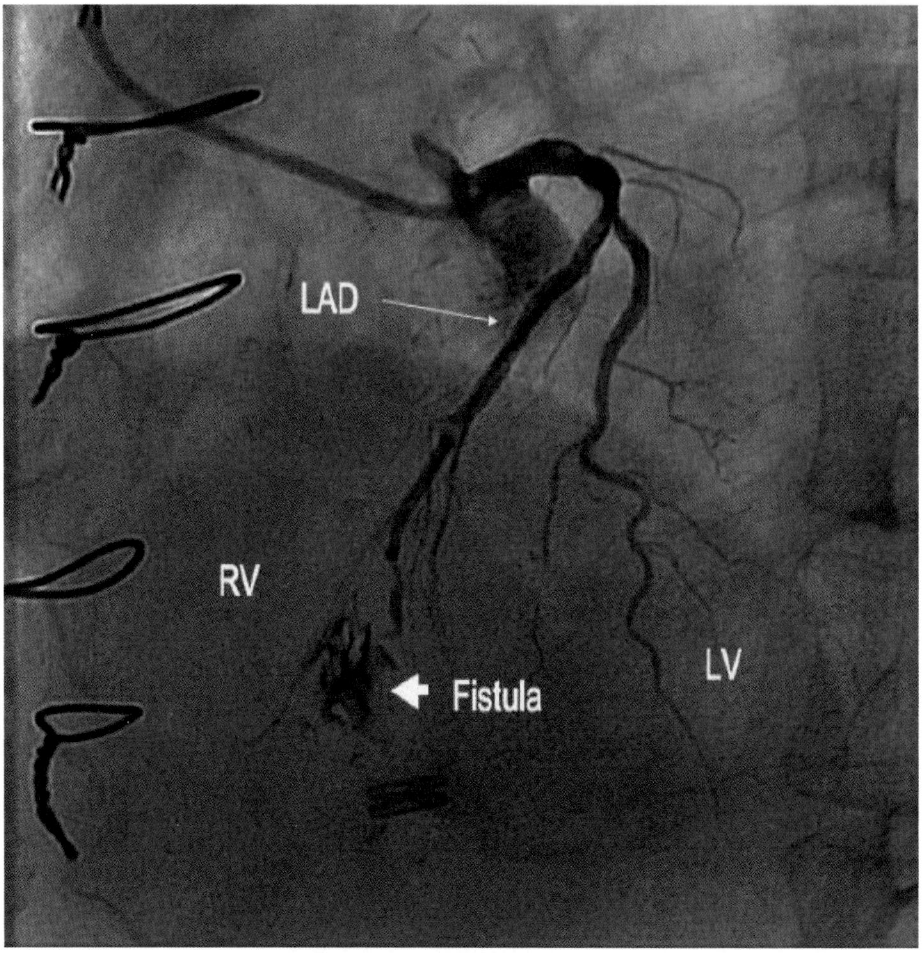

Figure 18. Arteriogram of Left Anterior Descending Artery to RV fistula.

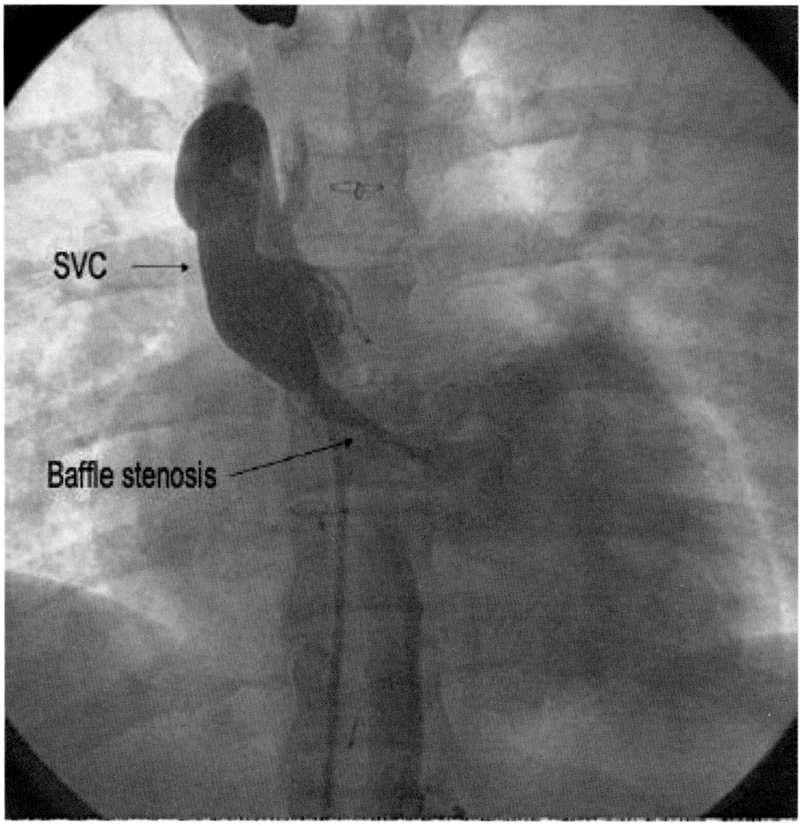

Figure 19. Arteriogram of repaired D-TGA with baffle stenosis.

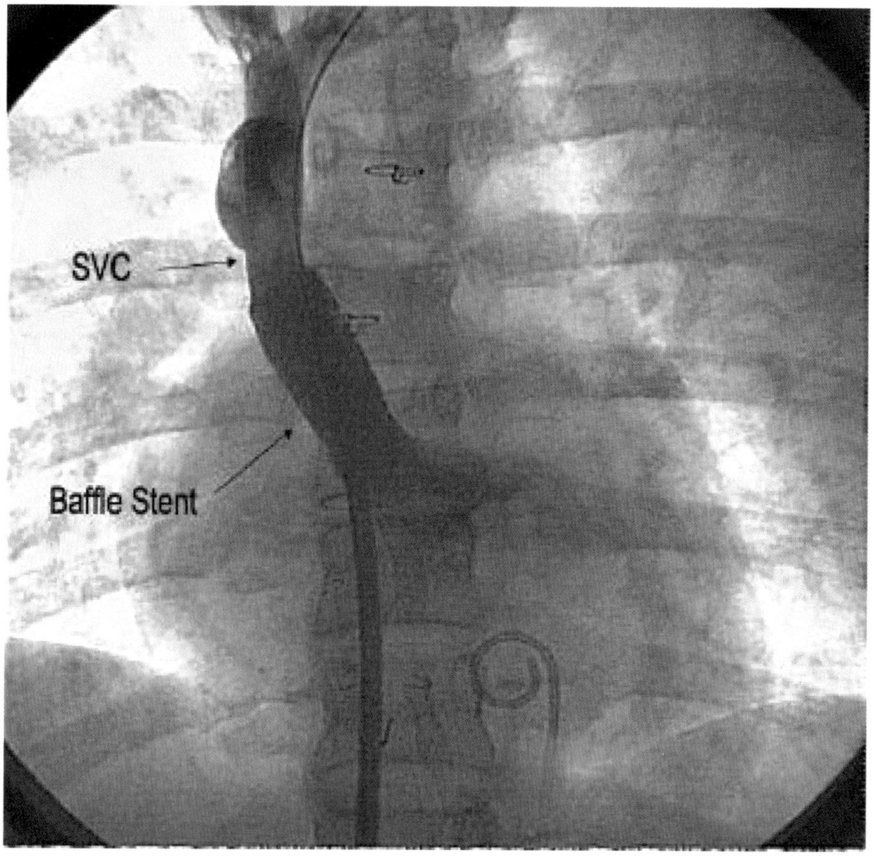

Figure 20. Arteriogram of repaired D-TGA with baffle stenosis s/p stenting.

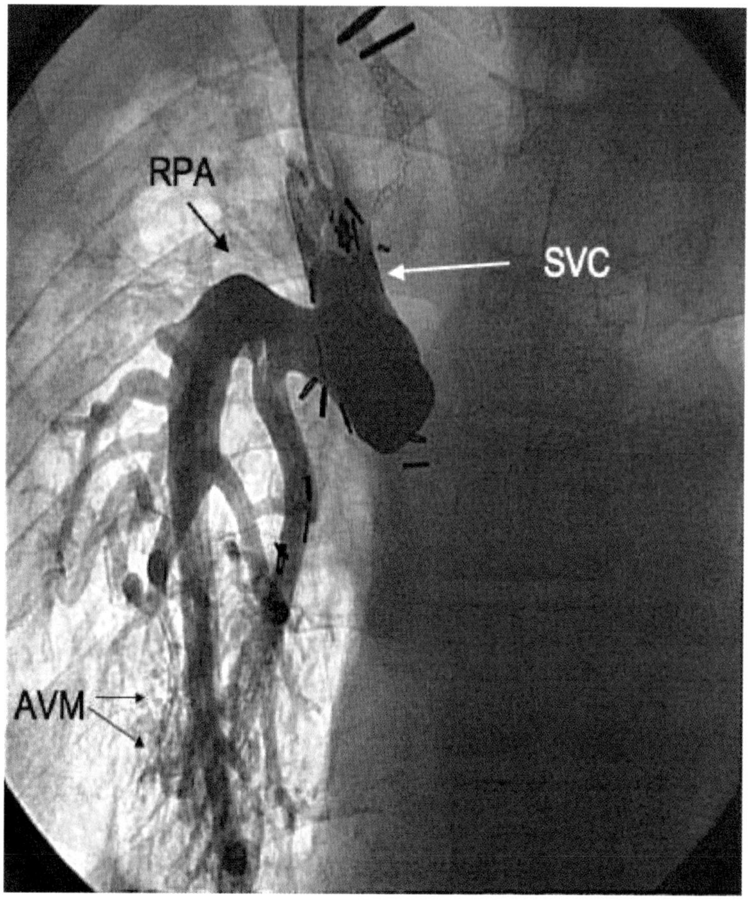

Figure 21. Arteriogram of a Superior Vena Cava to Right Pulmonary Artery shunt with associated arteriovenous malformations in the pulmonary arteries.

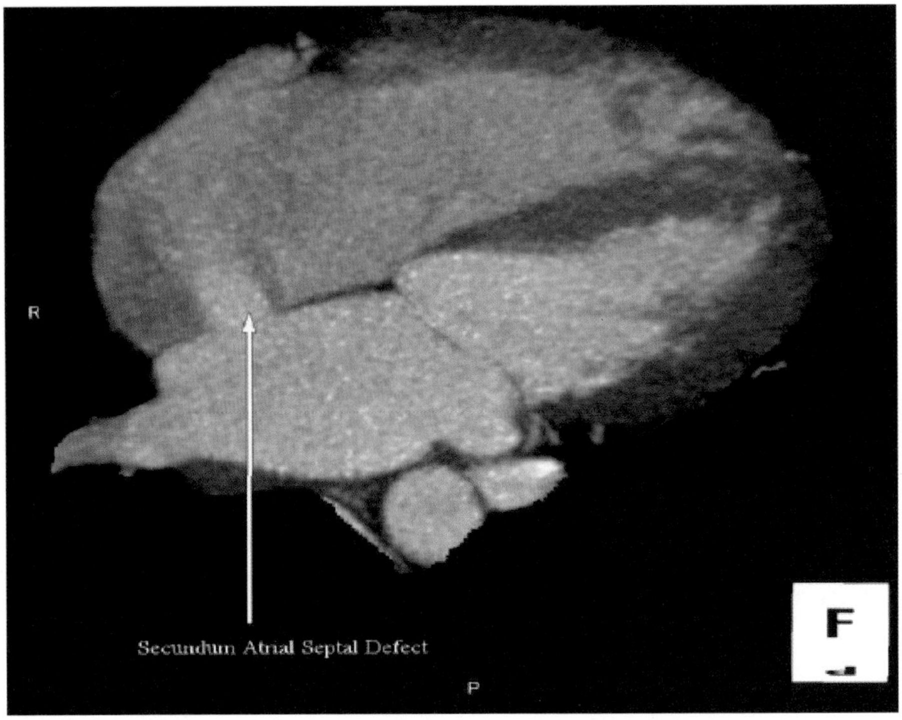

Figure 22. CT of secundum ASD.

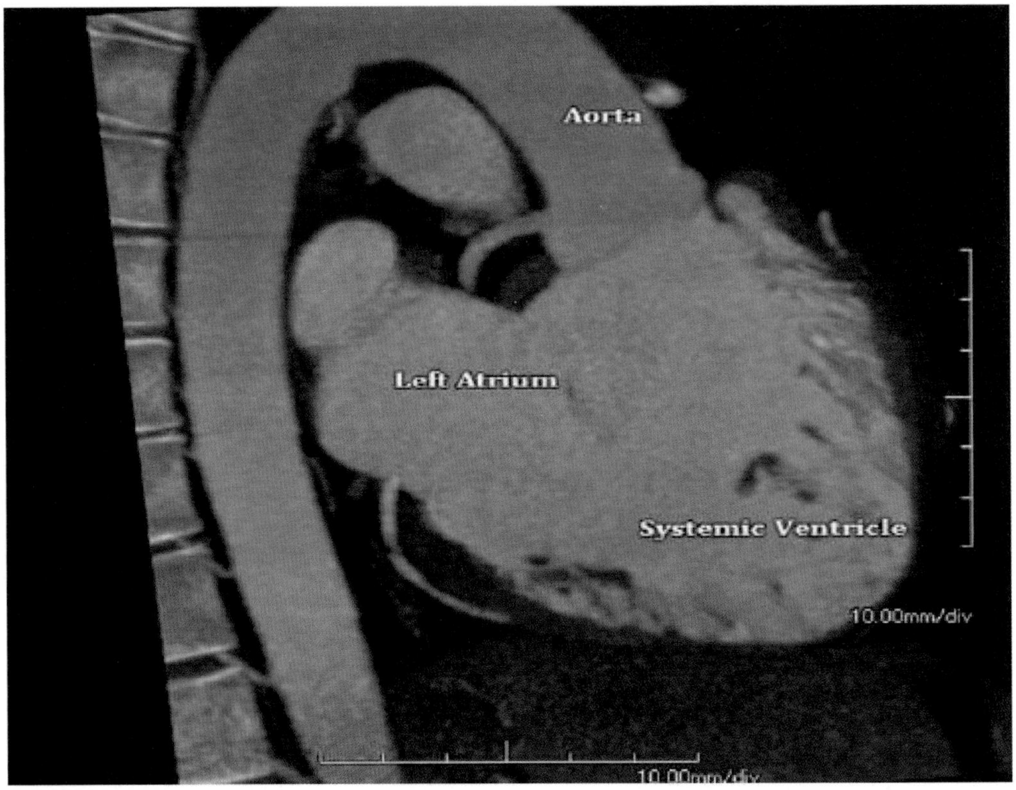

Figure 23. CT of CCTGA.

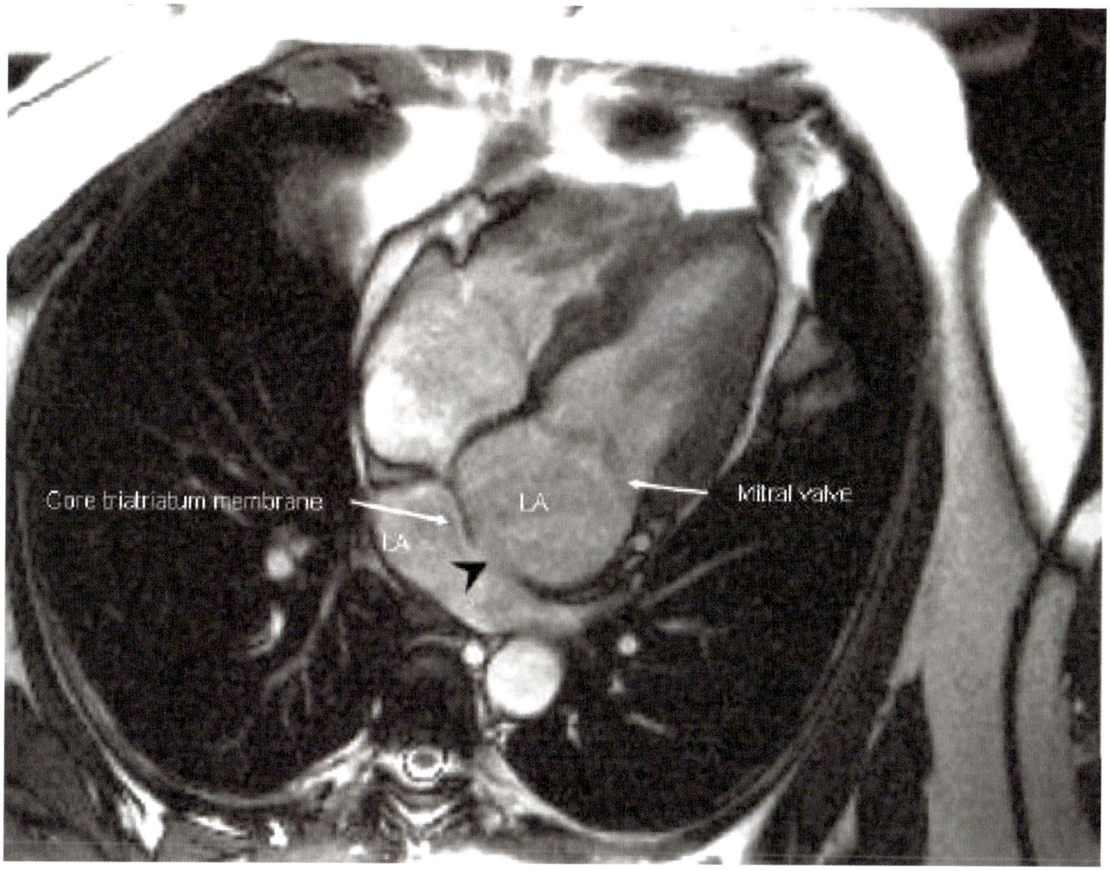

Figure 24. MRI of cor triatriatum.

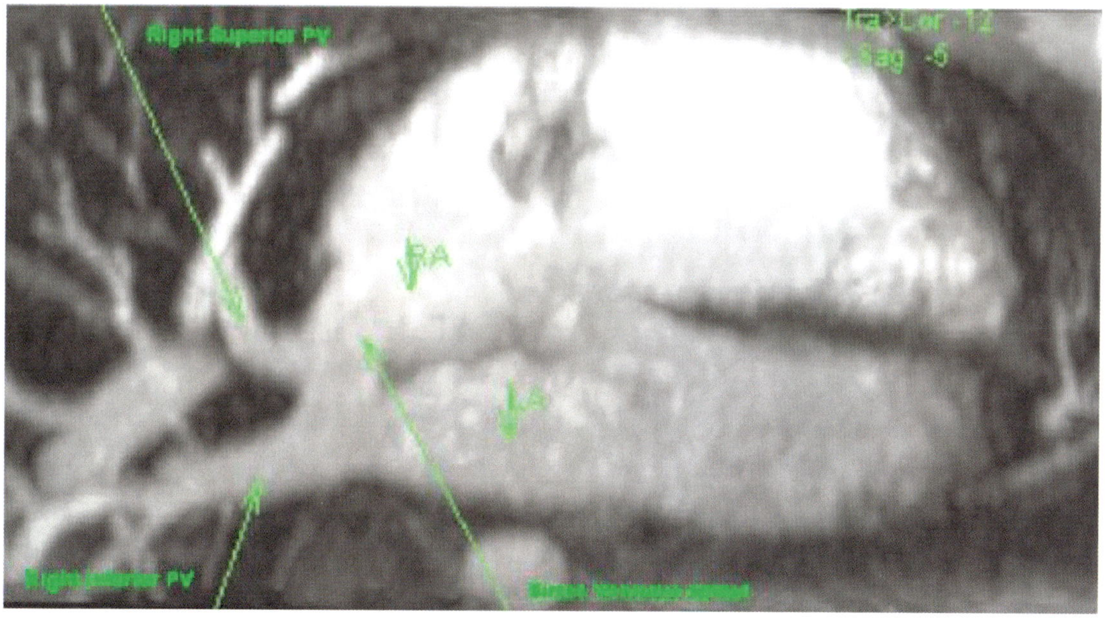

Figure 25. MRI of sinus venosus defect with partial anomalous venous return.

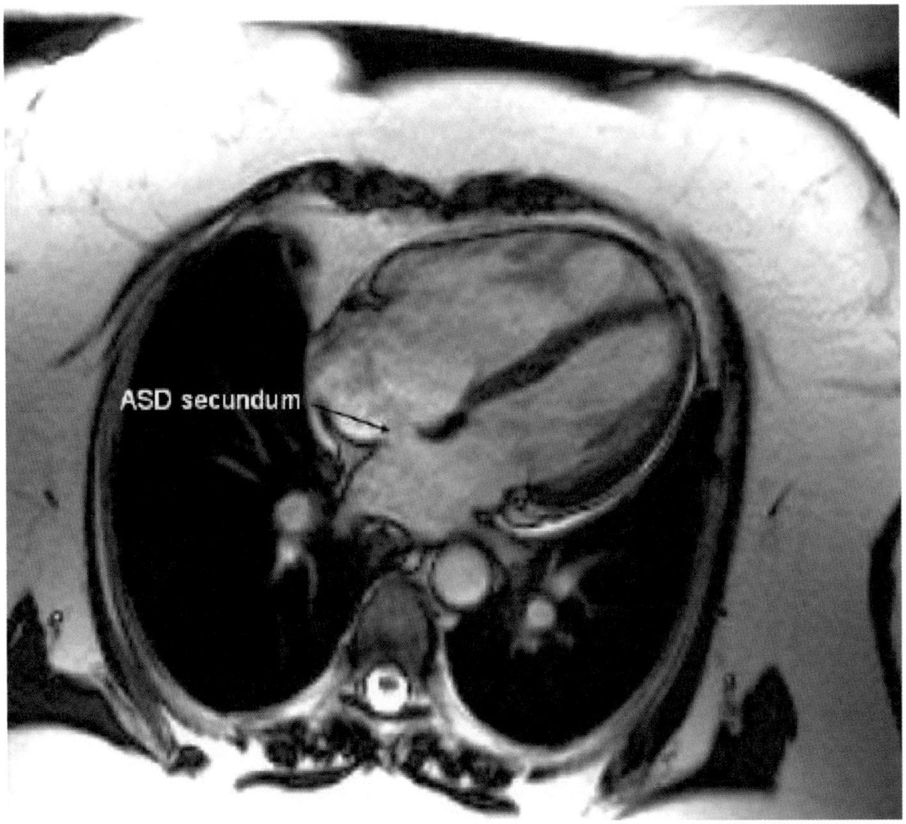

Figure 26. MRI of ASD Secundum Defect.

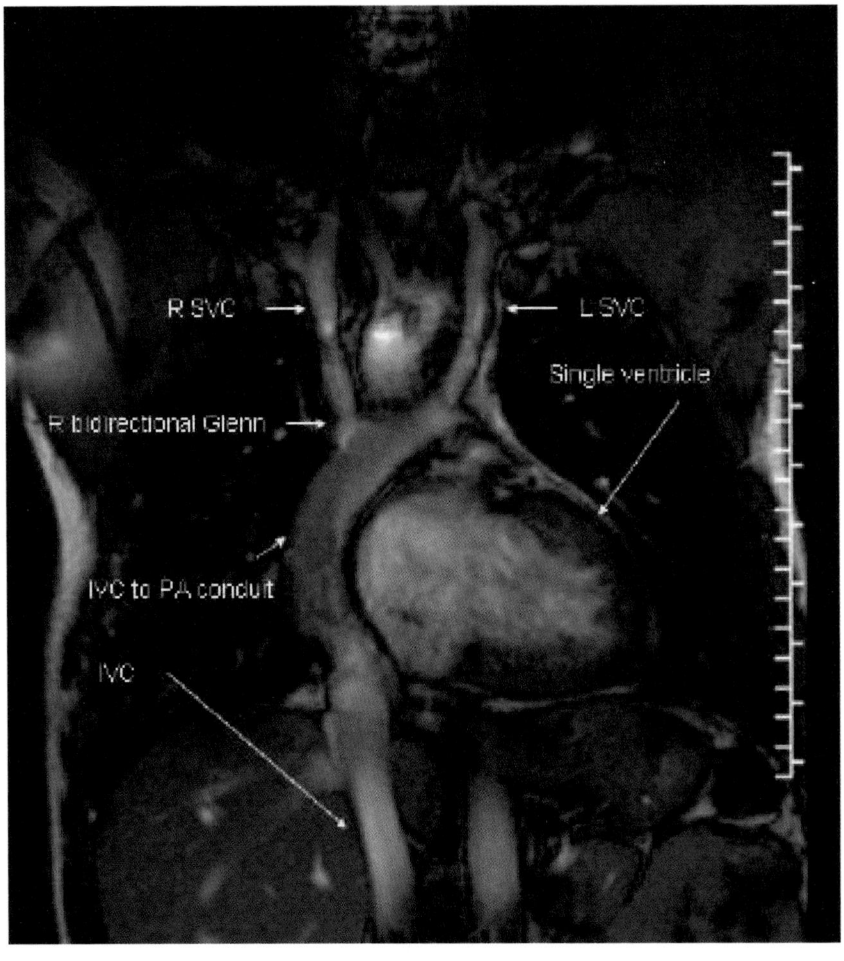

Figure 27a. MRI of Single Ventricle Physiology s/p Bidirectional Glenn.

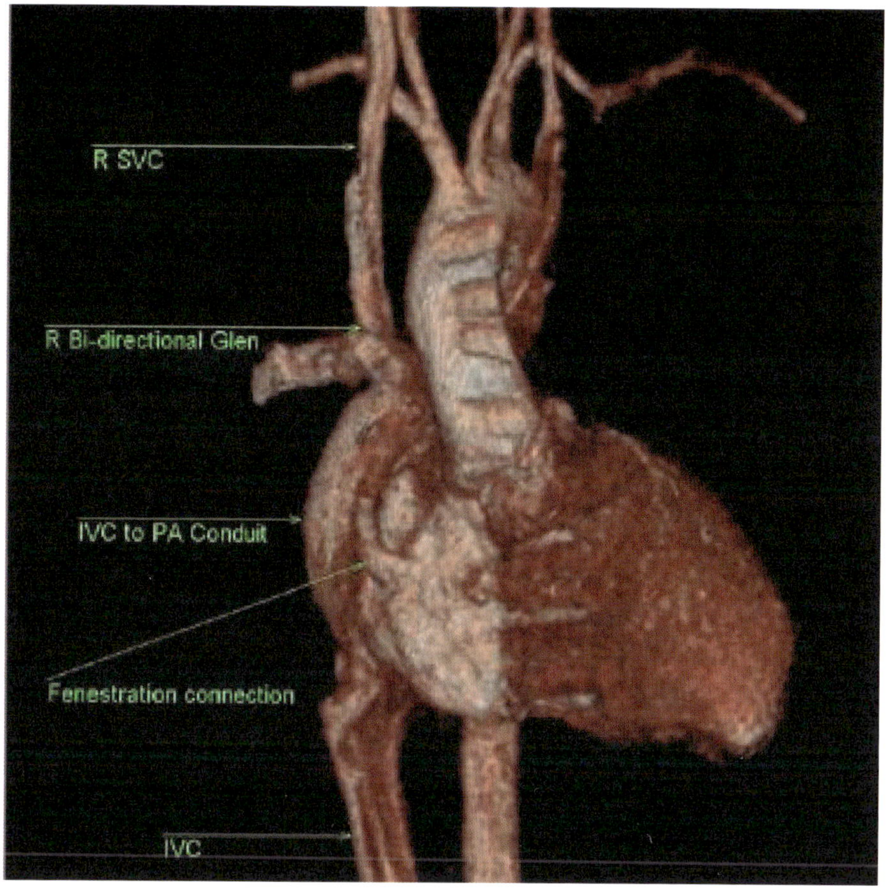

Figure 27b. MRI 3D reconstruction of Bidirectional Glenn.

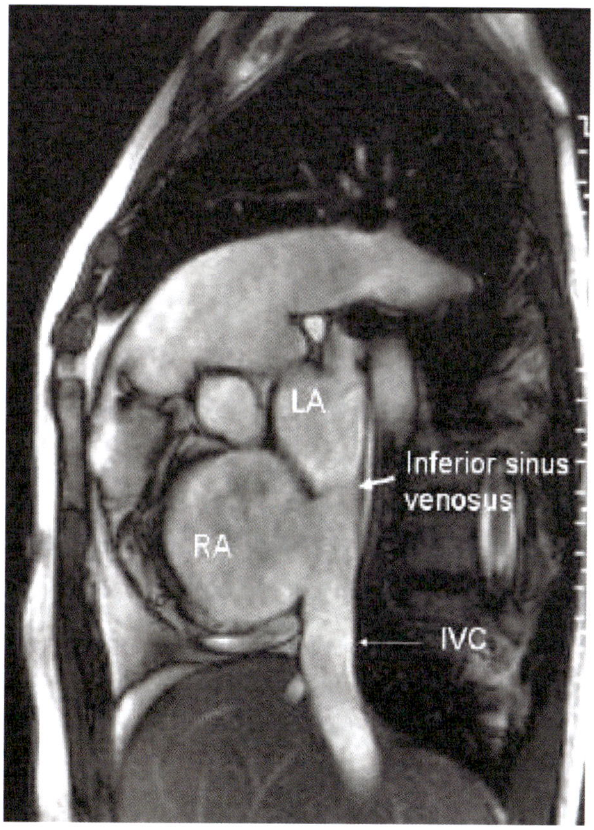

Figure 28. MRI of Inferior Sinus Venosus Defect.

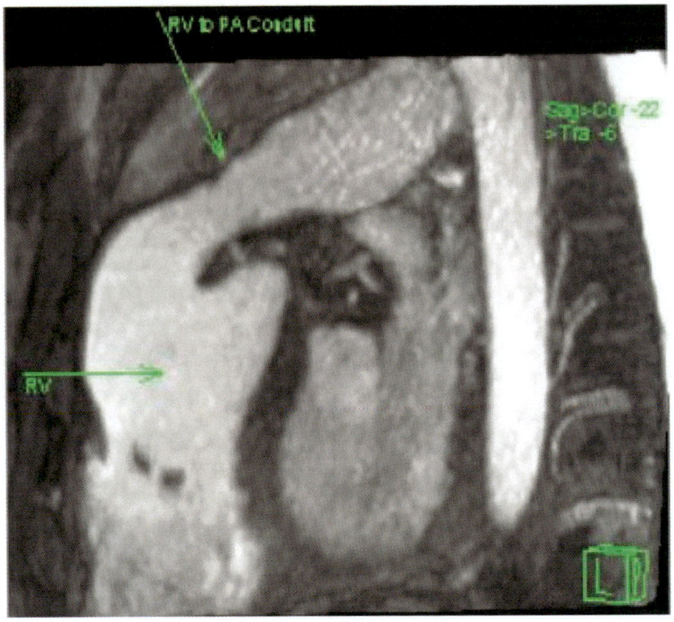

Figure 29. Tetralogy of Fallot with Severe Infundibular Stenosis.

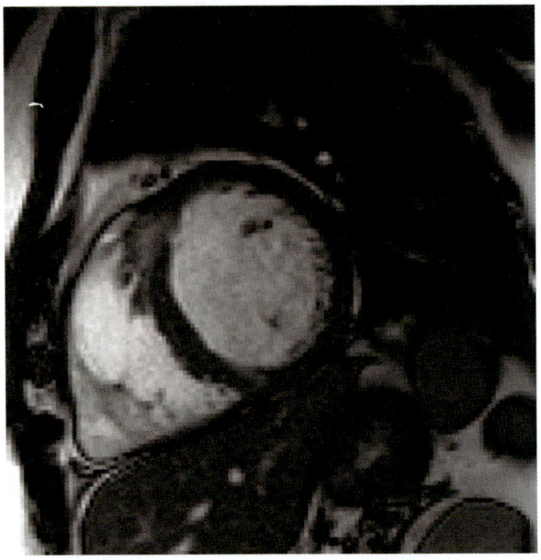

Figure 30. MRI of VSD.

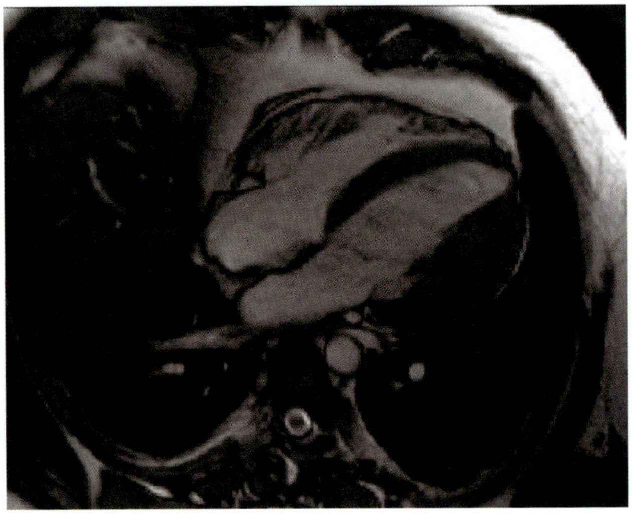

Figure 31a. MRI showing parachute mitral valve with single large papillary muscle.

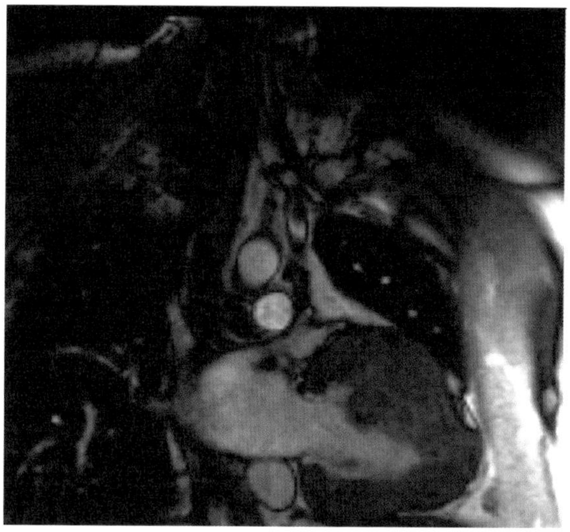

Figure 31b. Shone's Complex.

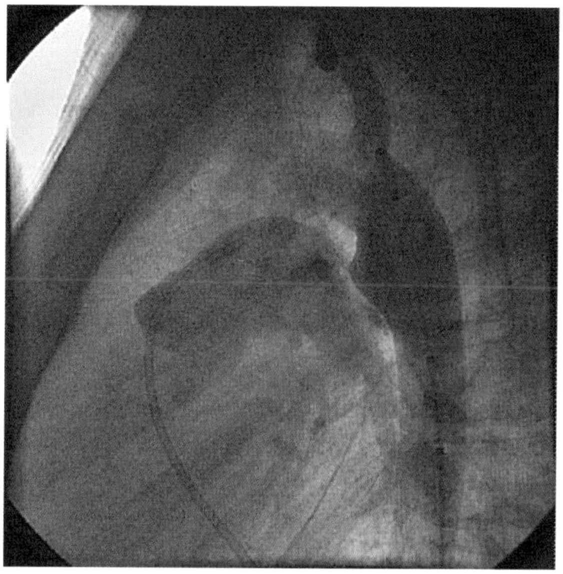

Figure 32a. Angiogram. PDA pre-closure.

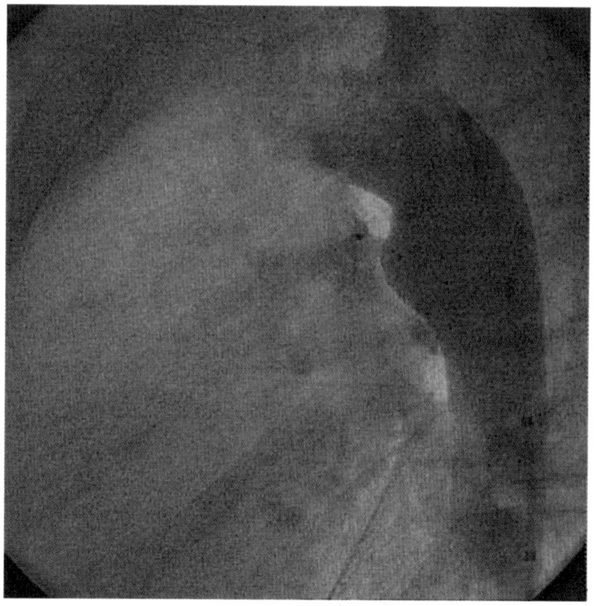

Figure 32b. Angiogram. PDA post-closure.

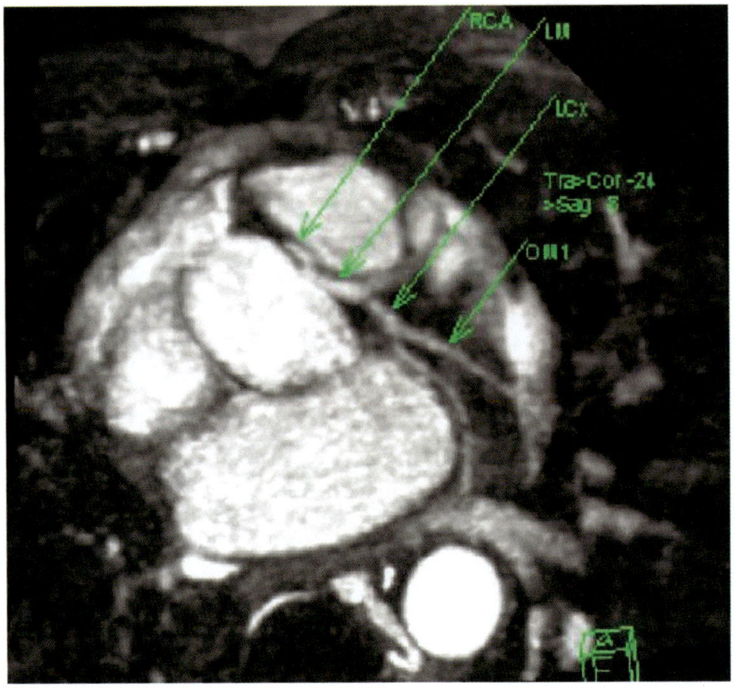

Figure 33. MRA showing anomalous coronary arteries with single origin of the RCA and left main coronary artery from the left coronary cusp.

Appendix B: 2008 ACC/AHA Guidelines for the Management of Adults with Congenital Heart Disease

SIZE OF TREATMENT EFFECT →

ESTIMATE OF CERTAINTY (PRECISION) OF TREATMENT EFFECT

	CLASS I *Benefit >>> Risk* Procedure/Treatment **SHOULD** be performed/administered	**CLASS IIa** *Benefit >> Risk* *Additional studies with focused objectives needed* **IT IS REASONABLE** to perform procedure/administer treatment	**CLASS IIb** *Benefit ≥ Risk* *Additional studies with broad objectives needed; additional registry data would be helpful* Procedure/Treatment **MAY BE CONSIDERED**	**CLASS III** *Risk ≥ Benefit* Procedure/Treatment should **NOT** be performed/administered **SINCE IT IS NOT HELPFUL AND MAY BE HARMFUL**
LEVEL A Multiple populations evaluated* Data derived from multiple randomized clinical trials or meta-analyses	■ Recommendation that procedure or treatment is useful/effective ■ Sufficient evidence from multiple randomized trials or meta-analyses	■ Recommendation in favor of treatment or procedure being useful/effective ■ Some conflicting evidence from multiple randomized trials or meta-analyses	■ Recommendation's usefulness/efficacy less well established ■ Greater conflicting evidence from multiple randomized trials or meta-analyses	■ Recommendation that procedure or treatment is not useful/effective and may be harmful ■ Sufficient evidence from multiple randomized trials or meta-analyses
LEVEL B Limited populations evaluated* Data derived from a single randomized trial or nonrandomized studies	■ Recommendation that procedure or treatment is useful/effective ■ Evidence from single randomized trial or nonrandomized studies	■ Recommendation in favor of treatment or procedure being useful/effective ■ Some conflicting evidence from single randomized trial or nonrandomized studies	■ Recommendation's usefulness/efficacy less well established ■ Greater conflicting evidence from single randomized trial or nonrandomized studies	■ Recommendation that procedure or treatment is not useful/effective and may be harmful ■ Evidence from single randomized trial or nonrandomized studies
LEVEL C Very limited populations evaluated* Only consensus opinion of experts, case studies, or standard of care	■ Recommendation that procedure or treatment is useful/effective ■ Only expert opinion, case studies, or standard of care	■ Recommendation in favor of treatment or procedure being useful/effective ■ Only diverging expert opinion, case studies, or standard of care	■ Recommendation's usefulness/efficacy less well established ■ Only diverging expert opinion, case studies, or standard of care	■ Recommendation that procedure or treatment is not useful/effective and may be harmful ■ Only expert opinion, case studies, or standard of care
Suggested phrases for writing recommendations†	should is recommended is indicated is useful/effective/beneficial	is reasonable can be useful/effective/beneficial is probably recommended or indicated	may/might be considered may/might be reasonable usefulness/effectiveness is unknown/unclear/uncertain or not well established	is not recommended is not indicated should not is not useful/effective/beneficial may be harmful

Figure 34. Applying Classification of Recommendations and Level of Evidence.

Table 1. Recommendations for Atrial Septal Defects

	Recommendation	Level of evidence
Recommendations for Medical Therapy	Cardioversion after appropriate anticoagulation is recommended to attempt restoration of the sinus rhythm if atrial fibrillation occurs	I:A
	Rate control and anticoagulation are recommended if sinus rhythm cannot be maintained by medical or interventional means.	I:A
Recommendations for Interventional and Surgical Therapy	Closure of an ASD either percutaneously or surgically is indicated for right atrial and RV enlargement with or without symptoms.	I:B
	A sinus venosus, coronary sinus, or primum ASD should be repaired surgically rather than by percutaneous closure.	I:B
	Surgeons with training and expertise in CHD should perform operations for various ASD closures	I:C
	Surgical closure of secundum ASD is reasonable when concomitant surgical repair/replacement of a tricuspid valve is considered or when the anatomy of the defect precludes the use of a percutaneous device.	IIa:C
	Closure of an ASD, either percutaneously or surgically, is reasonable in the presence of a Paradoxical embolism.	IIa:C
	Closure of an ASD, either percutaneously or surgically, is reasonable in the presence of documented orthodeoxia-platypnea	IIa:B
	Closure of an ASD, either percutaneously or surgically, may be considered in the presence of net left-to-right shunting, pulmonary artery pressure less than two thirds systemic levels, PVR less than two thirds systemic vascular resistance, or when responsive to either pulmonary vasodilator therapy or test occlusion of the defect (patients should be treated in conjunction with providers who have expertise in the management of pulmonary hypertensive syndromes).	IIb:C
	Concomitant Maze procedure may be considered for intermittent or chronic atrial tachyarrhythmias in adults with ASDs.	IIb:C
	Patients with severe irreversible PAH and no evidence of a left-to-right shunt should not undergo ASD closure.	III:B
Recommendations for Postintervention Follow-Up	Early postoperative symptoms of undue fever, fatigue, vomiting, chest pain, or abdominal pain may represent postpericardiotomy syndrome with tamponade and should prompt immediate evaluation with echocardiography.	I:C
	Annual clinical follow-up is recommended for patients postoperatively if their ASD was repaired as an adult and the following conditions persist or develop: a. PAH b. Atrial arrhythmias. c. RV or LV dysfunction. d. Coexisting valvular or other cardiac lesions.	I:C
	Evaluation for possible device migration, erosion, or other complications is recommended for patients 3 months to 1 year after device closure and periodically thereafter.	I:C
	Device erosion, which may present with chest pain or syncope, should warrant urgent evaluation.	I:C

Table 2. Recommendations for Ventricular Septal Defects

	Recommendation	Level of evidence
Recommendations for Cardiac Catheterization	Cardiac catheterization to assess the operability of adults with VSD and PAH should be performed in an ACHD regional center in collaboration with experts.	I:C
	Cardiac catheterization can be useful for adults with VSD in whom noninvasive data are inconclusive and further information is needed for management. Data to be obtained include the following: a. Quantification of shunting. b. Assessment of pulmonary pressure and resistance in patients with suspected PAH. Reversibility of PAH should be tested with various vasodilators.	IIa:B
	Cardiac catheterization can be useful for adults with VSD in whom noninvasive data are inconclusive and further information is needed for management. Data to be obtained include the following: c. Evaluation of other lesions such as AR and doublechambered right ventricle. d. Determination of whether multiple VSDs are present before surgery. e. Performance of coronary arteriography is indicated in patients at risk for coronary artery disease. f. VSD anatomy, especially if device closure is contemplated.	IIa:C
Recommendations for Medical Therapy	Pulmonary vasodilator therapy may be considered for adults with VSDs with progressive/severe pulmonary vascular disease	IIb:B
Recommendations for Surgical Ventricular Septal Defect Closure	Surgeons with training and expertise in CHD should perform VSD closure operations.	I:C
	Closure of a VSD is indicated when there is a Qp/Qs (pulmonary–to–systemic blood flow ratio) of 2.0 or more and clinical evidence of LV volume overload.	I:B
	Closure of a VSD is indicated when the patient has a history of IE.	I:C
	Closure of a VSD is reasonable when net left-to-right shunting is present at a Qp/Qs greater than 1.5 with pulmonary artery pressure less than two thirds of systemic pressure and PVR less than two thirds of systemic vascular resistance.	IIa:B
	Closure of a VSD is reasonable when net left-to-right shunting is present at a Qp/Qs greater than 1.5 in the presence of LV systolic or diastolic failure.	IIa:B
	VSD closure is not recommended in patients with severe irreversible PAH.	III:B
Recommendation for Interventional Catheterization	Device closure of a muscular VSD may be considered, especially if the VSD is remote from the tricuspid valve and the aorta, if the VSD is associated with severe left-sided heart chamber enlargement, or if there is PAH.	IIb:C
Recommendations for Surgical and Catheter Intervention Follow-Up	Adults with VSD with residual heart failure, shunts, PAH, AR, or RV outflow tract (RVOT) or LV outflow tract (LVOT) obstruction should be seen at least annually at an ACHD regional center.	I:C
	Adults with a small residual VSD and no other lesions should be seen every 3 to 5 years at an ACHD regional center.	I:C
Recommendations for Surgical and Catheter Intervention Follow-Up	Adults with device closure of a VSD should be followed up every 1 to 2 years at an ACHD center depending on the location of the VSD and other factors.	I:C

Table 3. Atrioventricular Septal Defect Recommendations

	Recommendation	Level of evidence
Recommendations for Cardiac Catheterization	Cardiac catheterization is reasonable to assess PAH and test vasoreactivity in patients with repaired or unrepaired AVSD.	IIa:B
Recommendations for Surgical Therapy	Surgeons with training and expertise in CHD should perform operations for AVSD.	I:C
	Surgical reoperation is recommended in adults with previously repaired AVSD with the following indications: a. Left AV valve repair or replacement for regurgitation or stenosis that causes symptoms, atrial or ventricular arrhythmias, a progressive increase in LV dimensions, or deterioration of LV function.	I:B
	b. LVOT obstruction with a mean gradient greater than 50mm Hg or peak instantaneous gradient greater than 70mm Hg, or a gradient less than 50 mm Hg in association with significant mitral regurgitation or AR.	I:B
	c. Residual/recurrent ASD or VSD with significant left-toright shunting	I:B

Table 4. Patent Ductus Arteriosus

	Recommendation	Level of evidence
Recommendations for Evaluation of the Unoperated Patient	Definitive diagnosis of PDA should be based on visualization by imaging techniques and demonstrations of the shunting across the defect (with or without evidence of clinically significant LV volume overload).	I:C
	Diagnostic cardiac catheterization is not indicated for uncomplicated PDA with adequate noninvasive imaging.	III:B
	Maximal exercise testing is not recommended in PDA with significant PAH.	III:B
Recommendations for Medical Therapy	Routine follow-up is recommended for patients with a small PDA without evidence of left-sided heart volume overload. Follow-up is recommended every 3 to 5 years for patients with a small PDA without evidence of left-heart volume overload.	I:C
	Endocarditis prophylaxis is not recommended for those with a repaired PDA without residual shunt.	III:C
Recommendations for Closure of Patent Ductus Arteriosus	Closure of a PDA either percutaneously or surgically is indicated for the following: a. Left atrial and/or LV enlargement or if PAH is present, or in the presence of net left-to-right shunting.	I:C
	b. Prior endarteritis.	I:C
	Careful evaluation and consultation with ACHD interventional cardiologists is recommended before surgical closure is selected as the method of repair for patients with a calcified PDA.	I:C
	Surgical repair, by a surgeon experienced in CHD surgery, is recommended when: a. The PDA is too large for device closure.	I:C
	It is reasonable to close an asymptomatic small PDA by catheter device.	IIa:C
	PDA closure is reasonable for patients with PAH with a net left-to-right shunt.	IIa:C
	PDA closure is not indicated for patients with PAH and net right-to-left shunt.	III:C

Table 5. Recommendations for the Evaluation of Unoperated Valvular Aortic Stenosis and Medical Therapy

	Recommendation	Level of evidence
Recommendations for Evaluation of the Unoperated Patient	Primary imaging and hemodynamic assessment of AS and aortic valve disease are recommended by echocardiography- Doppler to evaluate the presence and severity of AS or AR; LV size, function, and mass; and dimensions and anatomy of the ascending aorta and associated lesions.	I:B
	Echocardiography is recommended for reevaluation of patients with AS who experience a change in signs or symptoms and for assessment of changes in AS hemodynamics during pregnancy.	I:B
	In asymptomatic adolescents and young adults, echocardiography-Doppler is recommended yearly for AS with a mean Doppler gradient greater than 30 mm Hg or peak instantaneous gradient greater than 50 mm Hg and every 2 years for patients with lesser gradients.	I:C
	Cardiac catheterization is recommended when noninvasive measurements are inconclusive or discordant with clinical signs.	I:C
	Coronary angiography is recommended before aortic valve surgery for coronary angiography in adults at risk for coronary artery disease.	I:B
	Coronary angiography is recommended before a Ross procedure if noninvasive imaging of the coronary arteries is inadequate.	I:C
	A yearly ECG is recommended in young adults less than 30 years of age with mean Doppler gradients greater than 30 mm Hg or peak Doppler gradients greater than 50 mm Hg.	I:C
	An ECG is recommended every other year in young adults less than 30 years of age with mean Doppler gradients less than 30 mm Hg or peak Doppler gradients less than 50 mm Hg.	I:C
	In asymptomatic young adults less than 30 years of age, exercise stress testing is reasonable to determine exercise capability, symptoms, and blood pressure response.	IIa:C
	Exercise stress testing is reasonable for patients with a mean Doppler gradient greater than 30 mm Hg or peak Doppler gradient greater than 50 mm Hg if the patient is interested in athletic participation or if clinical findings differ from noninvasive measurements.	IIa:C
	Exercise stress testing is reasonable for the evaluation of an asymptomatic young adult with a mean Doppler gradient greater than 40 mm Hg or a peak Doppler gradient greater than 64 mm Hg or when the patient anticipates athletic participation or pregnancy.	IIa:C
	Dobutamine stress testing can be beneficial in the evaluation of a mild aortic valve gradient in the face of low LV ejection fraction and reduced cardiac output.	IIa:B
Recommendations for Evaluation of the Unoperated Patient	MRI/CT can be beneficial to add important information about the anatomy of the thoracic aorta.	IIa:C
	Exercise stress testing can be useful to evaluate blood pressure response or elicit exercise-induced symptoms in asymptomatic older adults with AS.	IIa:B
	Magnetic resonance angiography may be beneficial in quantifying AR when other data are ambiguous or borderline.	IIb:C
	Exercise stress testing should not be performed in symptomatic patients with AS or those with repolarization abnormality on ECG or systolic dysfunction on echocardiography.	III:C
Recommendations for Medical Therapy	It is reasonable to treat systemic hypertension in patients with AS while monitoring diastolic blood pressure to avoid reducing coronary perfusion.	IIa:C
	It is reasonable to administer beta blockers in patients with BAV and aortic root dilatation.	IIa:C
	It is reasonable to use long-term vasodilator therapy in patients with AR and systemic hypertension while carefully monitoring diastolic blood pressure to avoid reducing coronary perfusion.	IIa:C
	It may be reasonable to treat patients with BAV and risk factors for atherosclerosis with statins with the aim of ''slowing down degenerative changes in the aortic valve and preventing atherosclerosis.	IIb:C
	Vasodilator therapy is not indicated for long-term therapy in AR for the following: The asymptomatic patient with only mild to moderate AR and normal LV function.	III:B
	Vasodilator therapy is not indicated for long-term therapy in AR for the following: The asymptomatic patient with LV systolic dysfunction who is otherwise a candidate for aortic valve replacement (AVR).	III:B
	Vasodilator therapy is not indicated for long-term therapy in AR for the following: The asymptomatic patient with either LV systolic function or mild to moderate LV diastolic dysfunction who is otherwise a candidate for AVR.	III:C

Reproduced and Adapted with Permission
Circulation. 2008;118:e714-e833.

Table 6. Catheter and Surgical Intervention for Adults with Valvular Aortic Stenosis

	Recommendations	Level of evidence
Recommendations for Catheter Interventions for Adults with Aortic Valvular Stenosis	In young adults and others without significantly calcified aortic valves and no AR, aortic balloon valvotomy is indicated in the following patients: Those with symptoms of angina, syncope, dyspnea on exertion, and peak-to-peak gradients at catheterization greater than 50 mm Hg.	I:C
	In young adults and others without significantly calcified aortic valves and no AR, aortic balloon valvotomy is indicated in the following patients: Asymptomatic adolescents or young adults who demonstrate ST or T-wave abnormalities in the left precordial leads on ECG at rest or with exercise and a peak-to-peak catheter gradient greater than 60 mm Hg.	I:C
	Aortic balloon valvotomy is reasonable in the asymptomatic adolescent or young adult with AS and a peak-to-peak gradient on catheterization greater than 50 mm Hg when the patient is interested in playing competitive sports or becoming pregnant.	IIa:C
	Aortic balloon valvotomy may be considered as a bridge to surgery in hemodynamically unstable adults with AS, adults at high risk for AVR, or when AVR cannot be performed secondary to significant comorbidities.	IIb:C
	In older adults, aortic balloon valvotomy is not recommended as an alternative to AVR, although certain younger patients may be an exception and should be referred to a center with experience in aortic balloon valvuloplasties.	I:B
	In older adults, aortic balloon valvotomy is not recommended as an alternative to AVR, although certain younger patients may be an exception and should be referred to a center with experience in aortic balloon valvuloplasties.	III:B
	In asymptomatic adolescents and young adults, aortic balloon valvotomy should not be performed with a peak-to-peak gradient less than 40 mm Hg without symptoms or ECG changes.	III:B
Recommendations for Aortic Valve Repair/Replacement and Aortic Root Replacement	Aortic valvuloplasty, AVR, or Ross repair is indicated in patients with severe AS or chronic severe AR while they undergo coronary artery bypass grafting surgery on the aorta, or surgery on other heart valves.	I:C
	AVR is indicated for patients with severe AS and LV dysfunction (LV ejection fraction less than 50%).	I:C
	AVR is indicated in adolescents or young adults with severe AR who have: Development of symptoms.	I:C
Recommendations for Aortic Valve Repair/Replacement and Aortic Root Replacement	AVR is indicated in adolescents or young adults with severe AR who have: Development of persistent LV dysfunction (LV ejection fraction less than 50%) or progressive LV dilatation (LV end-diastolic diameter 4 standard deviations above normal).	I:C
	Surgery to repair or replace the ascending aorta in a patient with a BAV is recommended when the ascending aorta diameter is 5.0 cm or more or when there is progressive dilation at a rate greater than or equal to 5 mm per year	I:B
	AVR is reasonable for asymptomatic patients with severe AR and normal systolic function (ejection fraction greater than 50%) but with severe LV dilatation (LV end-diastolic diameter greater than 75 mm or end-systolic dimension greater than 55 mm*).	IIa:B
	Surgical aortic valve repair or replacement is reasonable in patients with moderate AS undergoing coronary artery bypass grafting or other cardiac or aortic root surgery.	IIa:B
	AVR may be considered for asymptomatic patients with any of the following indications: a. Severe AS and abnormal response to exercise. b. Evidence of rapid progression of AS or AR. c. Mild AS while undergoing coronary artery bypass grafting or other cardiac surgery and evidence of a calcific aortic valve. d. Extremely severe AS (aortic valve area less than 0.6 cm and/or mean Doppler systolic AV gradient greater than 60 mm Hg) in an otherwise good operative candidate. e. Moderate AR undergoing coronary artery bypass grafting or other cardiac surgery. f. Severe AR with rapidly progressive LV dilation, when the degree of LV dilation exceeds an end-diastolic dimension of 70 mm or end-systolic dimension of 50 mm, with declining exercise tolerance, or with abnormal hemodynamic response to exercise.	IIb:C

Reproduced and Adapted with Permission
Circulation. 2008;118:e714-e833.

	Recommendations	**Level of evidence**
Recommendations for Aortic Valve Repair/Replacement and Aortic Root Replacement	Surgical repair may be considered in adults with AS or AR and concomitant ascending aortic dilatation (ascending aorta diameter greater than 4.5 cm) coexisting with AS or AR.	IIb:B
	Early surgical repair may be considered in adults with the following indications: a. AS and a progressive increase in ascending aortic size. b. Mild AR if valve-sparing aortic root replacement is being considered.	IIb:C
	AVR is not useful for prevention of sudden death in asymptomatic adults with AS who have none of the findings listed under the Class IIa/IIb indications.	III:B
	AVR is not indicated in asymptomatic patients with AR who have normal LV size and function.	III:B
Recommendations for Key Issues to Evaluate and Follow-up	Lifelong cardiology follow-up is recommended for all patients with aortic valve disease (AS or AR) (operated or unoperated)	I:A
	Serial imaging assessment of aortic root anatomy is recommended for all patients with BAV, regardless of severity. The frequency of imaging would depend on the size of the aorta at initial assessment: if less than 40 mm, it should be reimaged approximately every 2 years; if greater than or equal to 40 mm, it should be reimaged yearly or more often as progression of root dilation warrants or whenever there is a change in clinical symptoms or findings.	I:B
	Prepregnancy counseling is recommended for women with AS who are contemplating pregnancy.	I:B
	Patient referral to a pediatric cardiologist experienced in fetal echocardiography is indicated in the second trimester of pregnancy to search for cardiac defects in the fetus.	I:C
	Women with BAV and ascending aorta diameter greater than 4.5 cm should be counseled about the high risks of pregnancy.	I:C
	Patients with moderate to severe AS should be counseled against competitive athletics and strenuous isometric exercise.	I:B
	Echocardiographic screening for the presence of BAV is recommended for first-degree relatives of patients with BAV.	I:B

Table 7. Recommendations for Subaortic Stenosis

	Recommendation	Level of evidence
Recommendations for Surgical Intervention	Surgical intervention is recommended for patients with SubAS and a peak instantaneous gradient of 50 mm Hg or a mean gradient of 30 mm Hg on echocardiography-Doppler.	I:C
	Surgical intervention is recommended for SubAS with less than a 50 mm Hg peak or less than a 30 mm Hg mean gradient and progressive AR and an LV dimension at end-systolic diameter of 50 mm or LV ejection fraction less than 55%.	I:C
	Surgical resection may be considered in patients with a mean gradient of 30 mm Hg, but careful follow-up is required to detect progression of stenosis or AR.	IIb:C
	Surgical resection may be considered for patients with less than a 50 mm Hg peak gradient or less than a 30 mm Hg mean gradient in the following situations: a. When LV hypertrophy is present.	IIb:C
	Surgical resection may be considered for patients with less than a 50 mm Hg peak gradient or less than a 30 mm Hg mean gradient in the following situations: b. When pregnancy is being planned.	IIb:C
	Surgical resection may be considered for patients with less than a 50 mm Hg peak gradient or less than a 30 mm Hg mean gradient in the following situations: c. When the patient plans to engage in strenuous/competitive sports.	IIb:C
	Surgical intervention is not recommended to prevent AR for patients with SubAS if the patient has trivial LVOT obstruction or trivial to mild AR.	III:C
Recommendations for Key Issues to Evaluate and Follow-up	Lifelong cardiology follow-up, including evaluation by and/or consultation with a cardiologist with expertise in ACHD, is recommended for all patients with SubAS, repaired or not.	I:C
	The unoperated asymptomatic adult with stable LVOT obstruction due to SubAS and a mean gradient less than 30 mm Hg without LV hypertrophy or significant AR should be monitored at yearly intervals for increasing obstruction, the development or progression of AR, and the evaluation of systolic and diastolic LV function.	I:B
	Stress testing to determine exercise capability, symptoms, ECG changes or arrhythmias, or increase in LVOT gradient is reasonable in the presence of otherwise equivocal indications for intervention.	IIa:C

Table 8. Recommendations for Supravalvular Aortic Stenosis

	Recommendation	Level of evidence
Recommendations for Evaluation of the Unoperated Patient	TTE and/or TEE with Doppler and either MRI or CT should be performed to assess the anatomy of the LVOT, the ascending aorta, coronary artery anatomy and flow, and main and branch pulmonary artery anatomy and flow.	I:C
	Assessment of anatomy and flow in the proximal renal arteries is recommended in ACHD patients with supravalvular AS.	I:C
	Assessment of systolic and diastolic ventricular function is recommended in ACHD patients with supravalvular AS.	I:C
	Assessment of aortic and mitral valve anatomy and function is recommended in ACHD patients with supravalvular AS.	I:C
	Adults with a history or presence of supravalvular AS should be screened periodically for myocardial ischemia.	I:C
	Exercise testing, dobutamine stress testing, positron emission tomography, or stress sestamibi with adenosine studies can be useful to evaluate the adequacy of myocardial perfusion.	IIa:C

Recommendations for Interventional and Surgical Therapy	Operative intervention should be performed for patients with supravalvular LVOT obstruction (discrete or diffuse) with symptoms (i.e., angina, dyspnea, or syncope) and/or mean gradient greater than 50 mm Hg or peak instantaneous gradient by Doppler echocardiography greater than 70 mm Hg.	I:B
	Surgical repair is recommended for adults with lesser degrees of supravalvular LVOT obstruction and the following indications: a. Symptoms (ie, angina, dyspnea, or syncope).	I:B
	Surgical repair is recommended for adults with lesser degrees of supravalvular LVOT obstruction and the following indications: b. LV hypertrophy.	I:C
	Surgical repair is recommended for adults with lesser degrees of supravalvular LVOT obstruction and the following indications: c. Desire for greater degrees of exercise or a planned pregnancy.	I:C
Recommendations for Interventional and Surgical Therapy	Surgical repair is recommended for adults with lesser degrees of supravalvular LVOT obstruction and the following indications: d. LV systolic dysfunction.	I:C
	Interventions for coronary artery obstruction in patients with supravalvular AS should be performed in ACHD centers with demonstrated expertise in the interventional management of such patients.	I:C
Recommendations for Key Issues to Evaluate and Follow-up	Both operated and unoperated patients with SupraAS should be followed up annually at a regional ACHD center.	I:C
	Long-term psychosocial assessment and oversight, including the need for legal guardianship, are recommended for patients with Williams syndrome.	I:C

Table 9. Recommendations for Aortic Coarctation

	Recommendation	Level of evidence
Recommendations for Clinical Evaluation and Follow-up	Every patient with systemic arterial hypertension should have the brachial and femoral pulses palpated simultaneously to assess timing and amplitude evaluation to search for the "brachial-femoral delay" of significant aortic coarctation. Supine bilateral arm (brachial artery) blood pressures and prone right or left supine leg (popliteal artery) blood pressures should be measured to search for differential pressure.	I:C
	Initial imaging and hemodynamic evaluation by TTE, including suprasternal notch acoustic windows, is useful in suspected aortic coarctation.	I:B
	Every patient with coarctation (repaired or not) should have at least 1 cardiovascular MRI or CT scan for complete evaluation of the thoracic aorta and intracranial vessels.	I:B
Recommendations for Interventional and Surgical Treatment of Aortic Coarctation in Adults	Intervention for coarctation is recommended in the following circumstances: a. Peak-to-peak coarctation gradient greater than or equal to 20 mm Hg.	I:C
	Intervention for coarctation is recommended in the following circumstances: b. Peak-to-peak coarctation gradient less than 20 mm Hg in the presence of anatomic imaging evidence of significant coarctation with radiological evidence of significant collateral flow.	I:C
Recommendations for Interventional and Surgical Treatment of Aortic Coarctation in Adults	Choice of percutaneous catheter intervention versus surgical repair of native discrete coarctation should be determined by consultation with a team of ACHD cardiologists, interventionalists, and surgeons at an ACHD center.	I:C
	Percutaneous catheter intervention is indicated for recurrent, discrete coarctation and a peak-to-peak gradient of at least 20 mm Hg.	I:B
	Surgeons with training and expertise in CHD should perform operations for previously repaired coarctation and the following indications: a. Long recoarctation segment.	I:B
	Surgeons with training and expertise in CHD should perform operations for previously repaired coarctation and the following indications: b. Concomitant hypoplasia of the aortic arch.	I:B
	Stent placement for long-segment coarctation may be considered, but the usefulness is not well established, and the long-term efficacy and safety are unknown.	IIb:C
Recommendations for Key Issues to Evaluate and Follow-up	Lifelong cardiology follow-up is recommended for all patients with aortic coarctation (repaired or not), including an evaluation by or consultation with a cardiologist with expertise in ACHD.	I:C
	Patients who have had surgical repair of coarctation at the aorta or percutaneous intervention for coarctation of the aorta should have at least yearly follow-up.	I:C
	Even if the coarctation repair appears to be satisfactory, late postoperative thoracic aortic imaging should be performed to assess for aortic dilatation or aneurysm formation.	I:B
	Patients should be observed closely for the appearance or reappearance of resting or exercise-induced systemic arterial hypertension, which should be treated aggressively after recoarctation is excluded.	I:B
	Evaluation of the coarctation repair site by MRI/CT should be performed at intervals of 5 years or less, depending on the specific anatomic findings before and after repair.	I:C
	Routine exercise testing may be performed at intervals determined by consultation with the regional ACHD center.	IIb:C

Table 10. Recommendations for Right Ventricular Outflow Tract Obstruction: Valvular Pulmonic Stenosis

	Recommendation	**Level of evidence**
Recommendations for Evaluation of the Unoperated Patient	Two-dimensional echocardiography-Doppler, chest x-ray, and ECG are recommended for the initial evaluation of patients with valvular PS.	I:C
	A follow-up physical examination, echocardiography-Doppler, and ECG are recommended at 5-year intervals in the asymptomatic patient with a peak instantaneous valvular gradient by Doppler less than 30 mm Hg.	I:C
	A follow-up echocardiography-Doppler is recommended every 2 to 5 years in the asymptomatic patient with a peak instantaneous valvular gradient by Doppler greater than 30 mm Hg.	I:C
	Cardiac catheterization is unnecessary for diagnosis of valvular PS and should be used only when percutaneous catheter intervention is contemplated.	III:C
Recommendations for Intervention in Patients with Valvular Pulmonary Stenosis	Balloon valvotomy is recommended for asymptomatic patients with a domed pulmonary valve and a peak instantaneous Doppler gradient greater than 60 mm Hg or a mean Doppler gradient greater than 40 mm Hg (in association with less than moderate pulmonary valve regurgitation).	I:B
	Balloon valvotomy is recommended for symptomatic patients with a domed pulmonary valve and a peak instantaneous Doppler gradient greater than 50 mm Hg or a mean Doppler gradient greater than 30 mm Hg (in association with less than moderate pulmonary regurgitation).	I.C
	Surgical therapy is recommended for patients with severe PS and an associated hypoplastic pulmonary annulus, severe pulmonary regurgitation, subvalvular PS, or supravalvular PS. Surgery is also preferred for most dysplastic pulmonary valves and when there is associated severe TR or the need for a surgical Maze procedure.	I:C
	Surgeons with training and expertise in CHD should perform operations for the RVOT and pulmonary valve.	I:B
Recommendations for Intervention in Patients with Valvular Pulmonary Stenosis	Balloon valvotomy may be reasonable in asymptomatic patients with a dysplastic pulmonary valve and a peak instantaneous gradient by Doppler greater than 60 mm Hg or a mean Doppler gradient greater than 40 mm Hg.	IIb:C
	Balloon valvotomy may be reasonable in selected symptomatic patients with a dysplastic pulmonary valve and peak instantaneous gradient by Doppler greater than 50 mm Hg or a mean Doppler gradient greater than 30 mm Hg.	IIb:C
	Balloon valvotomy is not recommended for asymptomatic patients with a peak instantaneous gradient by Doppler less than 50 mm Hg in the presence of normal cardiac output.	III:C
	Balloon valvotomy is not recommended for symptomatic patients with PS and severe pulmonary regurgitation.	III:C
	Balloon valvotomy is not recommended for symptomatic patients with a peak instantaneous gradient by Doppler less than 30 mm Hg.	III:C
Recommendation for Clinical Evaluation and Follow-up After Intervention	Periodic clinical follow-up is recommended for all patients after surgical or balloon pulmonary valvotomy, with specific attention given to the degree of pulmonary regurgitation; RV pressure, size, and function; and TR. The frequency of follow-up should be determined by the severity of hemodynamic abnormalities but should be at least every 5 years.	I:C

Table 11. Recommendations for Right Ventricular Outflow Tract Obstruction: Supravalvular, Branch, and Peripheral Pulmonary Stenosis

	Recommendation	Level of evidence
Recommendations for Evaluation of Patients with Supravalvular, Branch, and Peripheral Pulmonary Stenosis	Patients with suspected supravalvular, branch, or peripheral PS should have baseline imaging with echocardiography-Doppler plus 1 of the following: MRI angiography, CT angiography, or contrast angiography.	I:C
	Once the diagnosis is established, follow-up echocardiography- Doppler to assess RV systolic pressure should be performed periodically, depending on severity.	I:C
Recommendations for Interventional Therapy in the Management of Branch and Peripheral Pulmonary Stenosis Patients with Valvular Pulmonary Stenosis	Percutaneous interventional therapy is recommended as the treatment of choice in the management of appropriate focal branch and/or peripheral pulmonary artery stenosis with greater than 50% diameter narrowing, an elevated RV systolic pressure greater than 50 mm Hg, and/or symptoms.	I:B
	In patients with the above indications for intervention, surgeons with training and expertise in CHD should perform operations for management of branch pulmonary artery stenosis not anatomically amenable to percutaneous interventional therapy.	I:B
Recommendations for Evaluation and Follow-up	Patients with peripheral PS should be followed up every 1 to 2 years, on the basis of severity, with a clinical evaluation and echocardiography-Doppler to evaluate RV systolic pressure and RV function.	I:C
	Discussion with a cardiac surgeon with expertise in CHD should take place before percutaneous peripheral pulmonary artery interventions are undertaken.	I:C

Table 12. Recommendations for Right-Sided Heart Obstruction Due to Stenotic Right Ventricular–Pulmonary Artery Conduits or Bioprosthetic Valves

	Recommendation	Level of evidence
Recommendation for Evaluation and Follow-up after Right Ventricular-Pulmonary Artery Conduit or Prosthetic Valve	After surgical relief of RVOT obstruction with a conduit or prosthetic valve, patients should be followed up on a 1- to 2-year basis with echocardiography-Doppler assessment of RV systolic pressure and function, as well as a measurement of the gradient across the RVOT.	I:C
Recommendations for Reintervention in Patients with Right Ventricular-Pulmonary Artery Conduit or Bioprosthetic Pulmonary Valve Stenosis	Surgeons with training and expertise in CHD should perform operations for patients with severe pulmonary prosthetic valve stenosis (peak gradient greater than 50 mm Hg) or conduit regurgitation and any of the following: a. Decreased exercise capacity. b. Depressed RV function. c. At least moderately enlarged RV end-diastolic size. d. At least moderate TR.	I:C
	Either surgical or percutaneous therapy can be useful in symptomatic patients with discrete RV–pulmonary artery conduit obstructive lesions with greater than 50% diameter narrowing or when a bioprosthetic pulmonary valve has a peak gradient by Doppler greater than 50 mm Hg or a mean gradient greater than 30 mm Hg.	IIa:C
	Either surgical or percutaneous therapy can be useful in asymptomatic patients when a pulmonary bioprosthetic valve has a peak Doppler gradient greater than 50 mm Hg.	IIa:C
	Surgical intervention may be considered preferable to percutaneous catheter intervention when an associated Maze procedure is being considered for the treatment of atrial arrhythmia.	IIb:C

Table 13. Recommendations for Double-Chambered Right Ventricle

	Recommendation	Level of evidence
Recommendations for Intervention in Patients with Double-Chambered Right Ventricle	Surgery is recommended for patients with a peak midventricular gradient by Doppler greater than 60 mm Hg or a mean Doppler gradient greater than 40 mm Hg, regardless of symptoms.	I:B
	Symptomatic patients with a peak midventricular gradient by Doppler greater than 50 mm Hg or a mean Doppler gradient greater than 30 mm Hg may be considered for surgical resection if no other cause of symptoms can be discerned.	IIb:C

Table 14. Recommendations for Coronary Artery Abnormalities

	Recommendation	Level of evidence
General Recommendations for Evaluation and Surgical Intervention	Any patient with CHD who has had coronary artery manipulation should be evaluated for coronary artery patency, function, and anatomic integrity at least once in adulthood.	I:C
	Surgeons with training and expertise in CHD should perform operations for the treatment of coronary artery anomalies.	I:C
Recommendations for Coronary Anomalies Associated With Supravalvular Aortic Stenosis	Adults with a history or presence of supravalvular AS should be screened every 1 or 2 years for myocardial ischemia.	I:C
	Interventions for coronary artery obstruction in patients with Supravalvular AS should be performed in ACHD centers with demonstrated expertise in the interventional management of these patients.	I:C
Recommendation for Coronary Anomalies Associated With Tetralogy of Fallot	Coronary artery anatomy should be determined before any intervention for RV outflow.	I:C
Recommendation for Coronary Anomalies Associated With Dextro-Transposition of the Great Arteries After Arterial Switch Operation	Adult survivors with dextro-TGA (d-TGA) after arterial switch operation (ASO) should have noninvasive ischemia testing every 3 to 5 years.	I:C
Recommendations for Congenital Coronary Anomalies of Ectopic Arterial Origin	The evaluation of individuals who have survived unexplained aborted sudden cardiac death or with unexplained lifethreatening arrhythmia, coronary ischemic symptoms, or LV dysfunction should include assessment of coronary artery origins and course.	I:B
Recommendations for Congenital Coronary Anomalies of Ectopic Arterial Origin	CT or magnetic resonance angiography is useful as the initial screening method in centers with expertise in such imaging.	I:B
	Surgical coronary revascularization should be performed in patients with any of the following: a. Anomalous left main coronary artery coursing between the aorta and pulmonary artery.	I:B
	Surgical coronary revascularization should be performed in patients with any of the following: b. Documented coronary ischemia due to coronary compression (when coursing between the great arteries or in intramural fashion).	I:B
	Surgical coronary revascularization should be performed in patients with any of the following: c. Anomalous origin of the right coronary artery between aorta and pulmonary artery with evidence of ischemia.	I:B
	Surgical coronary revascularization can be beneficial in the setting of documented vascular wall hypoplasia, coronary compression, or documented obstruction to coronary flow, regardless of inability to document coronary ischemia.	IIa:C
	Delineation of potential mechanisms of flow restriction *via* intravascular ultrasound can be beneficial in patients with documented anomalous coronary artery origin from the opposite sinus.	IIa:C
	Surgical coronary revascularization may be reasonable in patients with anomalous left anterior descending coronary artery coursing between the aorta and pulmonary artery.	IIb:C
Recommendations for Anomalous Left Coronary Artery From the Pulmonary Artery	In patients with an anomalous left coronary artery from the pulmonary artery (ALCAPA), reconstruction of a dual coronary artery supply should be performed. The surgery should be performed by surgeons with training and expertise in CHD at centers with expertise in the management of anomalous coronary artery origins.	I:C
	For adult survivors of ALCAPA repair, clinical evaluation with echocardiography and noninvasive stress testing is indicated every 3 to 5 years.	I:C

Table 15. Recommendations for Coronary Arteriovenous Fistula

	Recommendation	Level of evidence
Recommendations for Evaluation and Management	If a continuous murmur is present, its origin should be defined either by echocardiography, MRI, CT angiography, or cardiac catheterization.	I:C
	A large coronary arteriovenous fistula (CAVF), regardless of symptomatology, should be closed via either a transcatheter or surgical route after delineation of its course and its potential to fully obliterate the fistula.	I:C
	A small to moderate CAVF in the presence of documented myocardial ischemia, arrhythmia, otherwise unexplained ventricular systolic or diastolic dysfunction or enlargement, or endarteritis should be closed *via* either a transcatheter or surgical approach after delineation of its course and its potential to fully obliterate the fistula.	I:C
	Clinical follow-up with echocardiography every 3 to 5 years can be useful for patients with small, asymptomatic CAVF to exclude development of symptoms or arrhythmias or progression of size or chamber enlargement that might alter management.	IIa:C
	Patients with small, asymptomatic CAVF should not undergo closure of CAVF.	III:C
Recommendations for Management Strategies	Surgeons with training and expertise in CHD should perform operations for management of patients with CAVF.	I:C
	Transcatheter closure of CAVF should be performed only in centers with expertise in such procedures.	I:C
	Transcatheter delineation of CAVF course and access to distal drainage should be performed in all patients with audible continuous murmur and recognition of CAVF.	I:C

Table 16. Recommendations for Pulmonary Hypertension and Eisenmenger Physiology

	Recommendation	Level of evidence
Recommendations for Evaluation of the Patient with Pulmonary Arterial Hypertension	Care of adult patients with CHD-related PAH should be performed in centers that have shared expertise and training in both ACHD and PAH.	I:C
	The evaluation of all ACHD patients with suspected PAH should include noninvasive assessment of cardiovascular anatomy and potential shunting, as detailed below: a. Pulse oximetry, with and without administration of supplemental oxygen, as appropriate. b. Chest x-ray. c. ECG. d. Diagnostic cardiovascular imaging via TTE, TEE, MRI, or CT as appropriate. e. Complete blood count and nuclear lung scintigraphy.	I:C
	If PAH is identified but its causes are not fully recognized, additional testing should include the following: a. Pulmonary function tests with volumes and diffusion capacity (diffusing capacity of the lung for carbon monoxide). b. Pulmonary embolism–protocol CT with parenchymal lung windows. c. Additional testing as appropriate to rule out contributing causes of PAH. d. Cardiac catheterization at least once, with potential for vasodilator testing or anatomic intervention, at a center with expertise in catheterization, PAH, and management of CHD-PAH.	I:C
	It is reasonable to include a 6-minute walk test or similar nonmaximal cardiopulmonary exercise test as part of the functional assessment of patients with CHD-PAH.	IIa:C

(Table 16) Contd.....

	Recommendation	**Level of evidence**
Recommendations for Medical Therapy for Eisenmenger Physiology	It is recommended that patients with Eisenmenger syndrome avoid the following activities or exposures, which carry increased risks: Pregnancy. Iron deficiency.	I:B
	It is recommended that patients with Eisenmenger syndrome avoid the following activities or exposures, which carry increased risks: Dehydration. Moderate and severe strenuous exercise, particularly isometric exercise. e. Acute exposure to excessive heat (eg, hot tub or sauna). f. Chronic high-altitude exposure, because this causes further reduction in oxygen saturation and increased risk of altitude-related cardiopulmonary complications (particularly at an elevation greater than 5000 feet above sea level).	I:C
Recommendations for Medical Therapy for Eisenmenger Physiology	Patients with Eisenmenger syndrome should seek prompt therapy for arrhythmias and infections.	I:C
	Patients with Eisenmenger syndrome should have hemoglobin, platelet count, iron stores, creatinine, and uric acid assessed at least yearly.	I:C
	Patients with Eisenmenger syndrome should have assessment of digital oximetry, both with and without supplemental oxygen therapy, at least yearly. The presence of oxygen-responsive hypoxemia should be investigated further.	I:C
	Exclusion of air bubbles in intravenous tubing is recommended as essential during treatment of adults with Eisenmenger syndrome.	I:C
	Patients with Eisenmenger syndrome should undergo noncardiac surgery and cardiac catheterization only in centers with expertise in the care of such patients. In emergent or urgent situations in which transportation is not feasible, consultation with designated caregivers in centers with expertise in the care of patients with Eisenmenger syndrome should be performed and sustained throughout care.	I:C
	All medications given to patients with Eisenmenger physiology should undergo rigorous review for the potential to change systemic blood pressure, loading conditions, intravascular shunting, and renal or hepatic flow or function.	IIa:C
	Pulmonary vasodilator therapy can be beneficial for patients with Eisenmenger physiology because of the potential for improved quality of life.	IIa:C
Recommendations for Follow-up	Patients with CHD-related PAH should: a. Have coordinated care under the supervision of a trained CHD and PAH provider and be seen by such individuals at least yearly. b. Have yearly comprehensive evaluation of functional capacity and assessment of secondary complications. c. Discuss all medication changes or planned interventions with their CHD-related PAH caregiver.	I:C
	Endocardial pacing is not recommended in patients with CHDPAH with persistent intravascular shunting, and alternative access for pacing leads should be sought (the risks should be individualized)	III:B

Table 17. Recommendations for Tetralogy of Fallot

	Recommendation	Level of evidence
Recommendations for Evaluation and Follow-Up of the Repaired Patient	Patients with repaired tetralogy of Fallot should have at least annual follow-up with a cardiologist who has expertise in ACHD.	I:C
	Patients with tetralogy of Fallot should have echocardiographic examinations and/or MRIs performed by staff with expertise in ACHD.	I:C
	Screening for heritable causes of their condition (e.g, 22q11 deletion) should be offered to all patients with tetralogy of Fallot.	I:C
	Before pregnancy or if a genetic syndrome is identified, consultation with a geneticist should be arranged for patients with tetralogy of Fallot.	I:B
	Patients with unrepaired or palliated forms of tetralogy should have a formal evaluation at an ACHD center regarding suitability for repair.	I:B
Recommendation for Imaging	Comprehensive echocardiographic imaging should be performed in a regional ACHD center to evaluate the anatomy and hemodynamics in patients with repaired tetralogy of Fallot.	I:B
Recommendations for Diagnostic and Interventional Catheterization for Adults With Tetralogy of Fallot	Catheterization of adults with tetralogy of Fallot should be performed in regional centers with expertise in ACHD.	I:C
	Coronary artery delineation should be performed before any intervention for the RVOT.	I:C
	Interventional catheterization in an ACHD center is indicated for patients with previously repaired tetralogy of Fallot with the following indications: a. To eliminate residual native or palliative systemic–pulmonary artery shunts. b. To manage coronary artery disease.	I:B
	Interventional catheterization in an ACHD center is reasonable in patients with repaired tetralogy of Fallot to eliminate a residual ASD or VSD with a left-to-right shunt greater than 1.5:1 if it is in an appropriate anatomic location.	IIa:C
	In adults with repaired tetralogy of Fallot, catheterization may be considered to better define potentially treatable causes of otherwise unexplained LV or RV dysfunction, fluid retention, chest pain, or cyanosis. In these circumstances, transcatheter interventions may include: a. Elimination of residual shunts or aortopulmonary collateral vessels. b. Elimination of additional muscular or patch-margin VSD.	IIb:C
Recommendations for Diagnostic and Interventional Catheterization for Adults With Tetralogy of Fallot	In adults with repaired tetralogy of Fallot, catheterization may be considered to better define potentially treatable causes of otherwise unexplained LV or RV dysfunction, fluid retention, chest pain, or cyanosis. In these circumstances, transcatheter interventions may include: c. Dilation (with or without stent implantation) of RVOT obstruction. d. Elimination of residual ASD.	IIb:B
Recommendations for Surgery for Adults With Previous Repair of Tetralogy of Fallot	Surgeons with training and expertise in CHD should perform operations in adults with previous repair of tetralogy of Fallot.	I:C
	Pulmonary valve replacement is indicated for severe pulmonary regurgitation and symptoms or decreased exercise tolerance.	I:B
	Coronary artery anatomy, specifically the possibility of an anomalous anterior descending coronary artery across the RVOT, should be ascertained before operative intervention.	I:C
	Pulmonary valve replacement is reasonable in adults with previous tetralogy of Fallot, severe pulmonary regurgitation, and any of the following: a. Moderate to severe RV dysfunction. b. Moderate to severe RV enlargement.	IIa:B

Reproduced and Adapted with Permission
Circulation. 2008;118:e714-e833.

(Table 17) Contd.....

	Recommendation	**Level of evidence**
Recommendations for Surgery for Adults With Previous Repair of Tetralogy of Fallot	Pulmonary valve replacement is reasonable in adults with previous tetralogy of Fallot, severe pulmonary regurgitation, and any of the following: c. Development of symptomatic or sustained atrial and/or ventricular arrhythmias. d. Moderate to severe TR.	IIa:C
	Collaboration between ACHD surgeons and ACHD interventional cardiologists, which may include preoperative stenting, intraoperative stenting, or intraoperative patch angioplasty, is reasonable to determine the most feasible treatment for pulmonary artery stenosis.	IIa:C
	Surgery is reasonable in adults with prior repair of tetralogy of Fallot and residual RVOT obstruction (valvular or subvalvular) and any of the following indications: a. Residual RVOT obstruction (valvular or subvalvular) with peak instantaneous echocardiography gradient greater than 50 mm Hg. b. Residual RVOT obstruction (valvular or subvalvular) with RV/LV pressure ratio greater than 0.7. c. Residual RVOT obstruction (valvular or subvalvular) with progressive and/or severe dilatation of the right ventricle with dysfunction. d. Severe AR with associated symptoms or more than mild LV dysfunction. e. A combination of multiple residual lesions (eg, VSD and RVOT obstruction) leading to RV enlargement or reduced RV function.	IIa:C
Recommendations for Surgery for Adults With Previous Repair of Tetralogy of Fallot	Surgery is reasonable in adults with prior repair of tetralogy of Fallot and residual RVOT obstruction (valvular or subvalvular) and any of the following indications: f. Residual VSD with a left-to-right shunt greater than 1.5:1. (*Level of Evidence: B*)	IIa:B
Recommendations for Arrhythmias: Pacemaker and Electrophysiology Testing	Annual surveillance with history, ECG, assessment of RV function, and periodic exercise testing is recommended for patients with pacemakers/automatic implantable cardioverter defibrillators.	I:C
	Periodic Holter monitoring can be beneficial as part of routine follow-up. The frequency should be individualized depending on the hemodynamics and clinical suspicion of arrhythmia.	IIa:C
	Electrophysiology testing in an ACHD center may be reasonable to define suspected arrhythmias in adults with tetralogy of Fallot.	IIb:C

Table 18. Recommendations for Dextro-Transposition of the Great Arteries

	Recommendation	Level of evidence
Recommendation for Evaluation of the Operated Patient With Dextro-Transposition of the Great Arteries	Patients with repaired d-TGA should have annual follow-up with a cardiologist who has expertise in the management of ACHD patients.	I:C
Recommendations for Imaging for d-TGA after Atrial Baffle Procedure	In patients with d-TGA repaired by atrial baffle procedure, comprehensive echocardiographic imaging should be performed in a regional ACHD center to evaluate the anatomy and hemodynamics.	I:B
	Additional imaging with TEE, CT, or MRI, as appropriate, should be performed in a regional ACHD center to evaluate the great arteries and veins, as well as ventricular function, in patients with prior atrial baffle repair of d-TGA.	I:B
	Echocardiography contrast injection with agitated saline can be useful to evaluate baffle anatomy and shunting in patients with previously repaired d-TGA after atrial baffle.	IIa:B
	TEE can be effective for more detailed baffle evaluation for patients with d-TGA.	IIa:B
Recommendations for Imaging for d-TGA after Arterial Switch Operation	Comprehensive echocardiographic imaging to evaluate the anatomy and hemodynamics in patients with d-TGA and prior ASO repair should be performed at least every 2 years at a center with expertise in ACHD.	I:C
	After prior ASO repair for d-TGA, all adults should have at least 1 evaluation of coronary artery patency. Coronary angiography should be performed if this cannot be established noninvasively.	I:C
	Periodic MRI or CT can be considered appropriate to evaluate the anatomy and hemodynamics in more detail	IIa:C
Recommendation for Cardiac Catheterization after Arterial Switch Operation	Coronary angiography is reasonable in all adults with d-TGA after ASO to rule out significant coronary artery obstruction.	IIa:C
Recommendations for Diagnostic Catheterization for Adults With Repaired Dextro-Transposition of the Great Arteries	Diagnostic catheterization of the adult with d-TGA should be performed in centers with expertise in the catheterization and management of ACHD patients.	I:C
Recommendations for Diagnostic Catheterization for Adults With Repaired Dextro-Transposition of the Great Arteries	For adults with d-TGA after atrial baffle procedure (Mustard or Senning), diagnostic catheterization can be beneficial to assist in the following: a. Assessment of baffle leak. b. Assessment of superior vena cava or inferior vena cava pathway obstruction. c. Assessment of pulmonary venous pathway obstruction. d. Suspected myocardial ischemia or unexplained systemic RV dysfunction. e. Significant LV outflow obstruction at any level (LV pressure greater than 50% of systemic levels, or less in the setting of RV dysfunction).	IIa:B
	For adults with d-TGA after atrial baffle procedure (Mustard or Senning), diagnostic catheterization can be beneficial to assist in the following: f. Hemodynamic assessment. g. Assessment of PAH, with potential for vasodilator testing.	IIa:C
	For adults with d-TGA, VSD, and PS, after Rastelli-type repair, diagnostic catheterization can be beneficial to assist in the following: a. Coronary artery delineation before any intervention for RVOT obstruction. b. Assessment of residual VSD. c. Assessment of PAH, with potential for vasodilator testing. d. Assessment of subaortic obstruction across the left ventricle–to–aorta tunnel.	IIa:C

(Table 18) Contd.....

	Recommendation	**Level of evidence**
Recommendations for Interventional Catheterization for Adults With Dextro-Transposition of the Great Arteries	Interventional catheterization of the adult with d-TGA can be performed in centers with expertise in the catheterization and management of ACHD patients.	IIa:C
	For adults with d-TGA after atrial baffle procedure (Mustard or Senning), interventional catheterization can be beneficial to assist in the following: a. Occlusion of baffle leak. b. Dilation or stenting of superior vena cava or inferior vena cava pathway obstruction. c. Dilation or stenting of pulmonary venous pathway obstruction.	IIa:B
	For adults with d-TGA after Arterial Switch Operation, interventional catheterization can be beneficial to assist in dilation or stenting of supravalvular and branch pulmonary artery stenosis.	IIa:B
	For adults with d-TGA, VSD, and PS, after Rastelli-type repair, interventional catheterization can be beneficial to assist in the following: a. Dilation with or without stent implantation of conduit obstruction (RV pressure greater than 50% of systemic levels, or peak-to-peak gradient greater than 30 mm Hg; these indications may be lessened in the setting of RV dysfunction). b. Device closure of residual VSD.	IIa:C
Recommendations for Surgical Interventions After Atrial Baffle Procedure	Surgeons with training and expertise in CHD should perform operations in patients with d-TGA and the following indications: a. Moderate to severe systemic (morphological tricuspid) AV valve regurgitation without significant ventricular dysfunction. b. Baffle leak with left-to-right shunt greater than 1.5:1, right-to-left shunt with arterial desaturation at rest or with exercise, symptoms, and progressive ventricular enlargement that is not amenable to device intervention. c. Superior vena cava or inferior vena cava obstruction not amenable to percutaneous treatment. d. Pulmonary venous pathway obstruction not amenable to percutaneous intervention. e. Symptomatic severe subpulmonary stenosis.	I:B
Recommendations for Surgical Interventions After Arterial Switch Operation	It is recommended that surgery be performed in patients after the ASO with the following indications: a. RVOT obstruction peak-to-peak gradient greater than 50 mm Hg or right ventricle/left ventricle pressure ratio greater than 0.7, not amenable or responsive to percutaneous treatment; lesser degrees of obstruction if pregnancy is planned, greater degrees of exercise are desired, or concomitant severe pulmonary regurgitation is present. b. Coronary artery abnormality with myocardial ischemia not amenable to percutaneous intervention. c. Severe neoaortic valve regurgitation. d. Severe neoaortic root dilatation (greater than 55 mm) after ASO. (This recommendation is based on data for other forms of degenerative aortic root aneurysms.)	I:C
Recommendations for Surgical Interventions After Rastelli Procedure	Reoperation for conduit and/or valve replacement after Rastelli repair of d-TGA is recommended in patients with the following indications: a. Conduit obstruction peak-to-peak gradient greater than 50 mm Hg. b. RV/LV pressure ratio greater than 0.7. (*Level of Evidence: C*) c. Lesser degrees of conduit obstruction if pregnancy is being planned or greater degrees of exercise are desired. d. Subaortic (baffle) obstruction (mean gradient greater than 50 mm Hg). e. Lesser degrees of subaortic baffle obstruction if LV hypertrophy is present, pregnancy is being planned, or greater degrees of exercise are desired. f. Presence of concomitant severe AR.	I:C
	Reoperation for conduit regurgitation after Rastelli repair of d-TGA is recommended in patients with severe conduit regurgitation and the following indications: a. Symptoms or declining exercise tolerance. b. Severely depressed RV function. c. Severe RV enlargement. d. Development/progression of atrial or ventricular arrhythmias. e. More than moderate TR.	I:C

Reproduced and Adapted with Permission
Circulation. 2008;118:e714-e833.

(Table 18) Contd.....

	Recommendation	Level of evidence
Recommendations for Surgical Interventions After Rastelli Procedure	Collaboration between surgeons and interventional cardiologists, which may include preoperative stenting, intraoperative stenting, or intraoperative patch angioplasty with or without conduit replacements, is recommended to determine the most feasible treatment for pulmonary artery stenosis.	I:C
Recommendations for Surgical Interventions After Rastelli Procedure	Surgical closure of residual VSD in adults after Rastelli repair of d-TGA is recommended with the following indicators: a. Qp/Qs greater than 1.5:1. b. Systolic pulmonary artery pressure greater than 50 mm Hg. c. RVOT obstruction (peak instantaneous gradient greater than 50 mm Hg). d. Pulmonary artery pressure less than two thirds of systemic pressure, or PVR less than two thirds of systemic vascular resistance, with a net left-to-right shunt of 1.5:1, or a decrease in pulmonary artery pressure with pulmonary vasodilators (oxygen, nitric oxide, or prostaglandins).	I:B
	Surgical closure of residual VSD in adults after Rastelli repair of d-TGA is recommended with the following indicators: e. Increasing LV size from volume overload. f. Decreasing RV function from pressure overload.	I:C
	Surgery is recommended after Rastelli repair of d-TGA in adults with branch pulmonary artery stenosis not amenable to percutaneous treatment.	I:C
	In the presence of a residual intracardiac shunt or significant systemic venous obstruction, permanent pacing, if indicated, should be performed with epicardial leads	I:B
	A concomitant Maze procedure can be effective for the treatment of intermittent or chronic atrial tachyarrhythmias in adults with d-TGA requiring reoperation for any reason.	IIa:B
Recommendations for Electrophysiology Testing/Pacing Issues in Dextro-Transposition of the Great Arteries	Clinicians should be mindful of the risk of sudden arrhythmic death among adults after atrial baffle repair of d-TGA. These events usually relate to ventricular tachycardia but may be caused in some cases by rapidly conducted IART or progressive AV block.	I:B
	Consultation with an electrophysiologist who is experienced with CHD is recommended to assist with treatment decisions.	I:B
	Pacemaker implantation is recommended for patients with d-TGA with either symptomatic sinus bradycardia or sick sinus syndrome.	I:B
	Routine surveillance with history, ECG, assessment of RV function, and periodic Holter monitoring can be beneficial as part of routine follow-up.	IIa:B

Table 19. Recommendations for Congenitally Corrected Transposition of the Great Arteries

	Recommendation	Level of evidence
Recommendations for Evaluation and Follow-up of Congenitally Corrected Transposition of the Great Arteries	All patients with CCTGA should have a regular follow-up with a cardiologist who has expertise in ACHD.	I:C
	Echocardiography-Doppler study and/or MRI should be performed yearly or at least every other year by staff trained in imaging complex CHD.	I:C
	The following diagnostic evaluations are recommended for patients with CCTGA: a. ECG. b. Chest x-ray. c. Echocardiography-Doppler study. d. MRI. e. Exercise testing.	I:C
Recommendations for Catheter Intervention	For patients with unrepaired CCTGA, cardiac catheterization can be effective to assess the following: Hemodynamic status in the setting of arrhythmia. b. Unexplained SV dysfunction, to define the degree of systemic AV valve regurgitation, degree of intracardiac shunting, and coronary artery anatomy. c. Unexplained volume retention or cyanosis, especially when noninvasive assessment of pulmonary outflow obstruction is limited.	IIa:C
Recommendations for Surgical Intervention	Surgeons with training and expertise in CHD should perform operations for patients with CCTGA for the following indications: a. Unrepaired CCTGA and severe AV valve regurgitation. b. Anatomic repair with atrial and arterial level switch/Rastelli repair in cases in which the left ventricle is functioning at systemic pressures. c. Simple VSD closure when the VSD is not favorable for LV-to-aorta baffling or is restrictive. d. LV–to–pulmonary artery conduit in rare cases with LV dysfunction and severe LV outflow obstruction. e. Evidence of moderate or progressive systemic AV valve regurgitation. f. Conduit obstruction with systemic or nearly systemic RV pressures and/or RV dysfunction after anatomic repair. g. Conduit obstruction and systemic or suprasystemic LV pressures in a patient with nonanatomic correction. h. Moderate or severe AR/neo-AR and onset of ventricular dysfunction or progressive ventricular dilatation.	I:B
Recommendations for Postoperative Care	Patients with prior repair of CCTGA should have regular follow-up with a cardiologist with expertise in ACHD.	I:C
	Echocardiography-Doppler study and/or MRI should be performed yearly or at least every other year by staff trained in imaging complex CHD.	I:C

Reproduced and Adapted with Permission
Circulation. 2008;118:e714-e833.

Table 20. Recommendations for Ebstein's Anomaly

	Recommendation	Level of evidence
Recommendation for Evaluation of Patients With Ebstein's Anomaly	All patients with Ebstein's anomaly should have periodic evaluation in a center with expertise in ACHD.	I:C
Recommendations for Diagnostic Tests	ECG, chest x-ray, and echocardiography-Doppler are recommended for the diagnostic evaluation of Ebstein's anomaly in adult patients.	I:C
	Pulse oximetry at rest and/or during exercise can be useful in the diagnostic evaluation of Ebstein's anomaly in adult patients.	IIa:C
	An electrophysiological study can be useful in the diagnostic evaluation of Ebstein's anomaly in adult patients if a supraventricular arrhythmia is documented or suspected (subsequent radiofrequency catheter ablation should be considered if clinically feasible).	IIa:C
	The following additional diagnostic tests can be useful for the comprehensive evaluation of Ebstein's anomaly in adult patients: a. Doppler TEE examination if the anatomic information is not provided by transthoracic imaging. b. Holter monitoring. c. Electrophysiological study for history or ECG evidence of accessory pathway(s). d. Coronary angiography, when surgical repair is planned, if there is a suspicion of coronary artery disease, and in men 35 years or older, premenopausal women 35 years or older who have coronary risk factors, and postmenopausal women.	IIa:B
Recommendation for Medical Therapy	Anticoagulation with warfarin is recommended for patients with Ebstein's anomaly with a history of paradoxical embolus or atrial fibrillation.	I:B
Recommendation for Catheter Interventions for Adults With Ebstein's Anomaly	Adults with Ebstein's anomaly should have catheterization performed at centers with expertise in catheterization and management of such patients.	I:C
Recommendation for Electrophysiology Testing/Pacing Issues in Ebstein's Anomaly	Catheter ablation can be beneficial for treatment of recurrent supraventricular tachycardia in some patients with Ebstein's anomaly.	IIa:B
Recommendations for Surgical Interventions	Surgeons with training and expertise in CHD should perform tricuspid valve repair or replacement with concomitant closure of an ASD, when present, for patients with Ebstein's anomaly with the following indications: a. Symptoms or deteriorating exercise capacity. b. Cyanosis (oxygen saturation less than 90%). c. Paradoxical embolism. d. Progressive cardiomegaly on chest x-ray. e. Progressive RV dilation or reduction of RV systolic function.	I:B
Recommendations for Surgical Interventions	Surgeons with training and expertise in CHD should perform concomitant arrhythmia surgery in patients with Ebstein's anomaly and the following indications: a. Appearance/progression of atrial and/or ventricular arrhythmias not amenable to percutaneous treatment. b. Ventricular preexcitation not successfully treated in the electrophysiology laboratory.	I:B
	Surgical rerepair or replacement of the tricuspid valve is recommended in adults with Ebstein's anomaly with the following indications: a. Symptoms, deteriorating exercise capacity, or New York Heart Association functional class III or IV. b. Severe TR after repair with progressive RV dilation, reduction of RV systolic function, or appearance/progression of atrial and/or ventricular arrhythmias. c. Bioprosthetic tricuspid valve dysfunction with significant mixed regurgitation and stenosis. d. Predominant bioprosthetic valve stenosis (mean gradient greater than 12 to 15 mm Hg). e. Operation can be considered earlier with lesser degrees of bioprosthetic stenosis with symptoms or decreased exercise tolerance.	I:B

Table 21. Recommendations for Tricuspid Atresia/Single Ventricle

	Recommendation	Level of evidence
Recommendation for Catheterization before Fontan Procedure	In the evaluation of hemodynamics to assess the potential for definitive palliation of unoperated or shunt-palliated adults with univentricular hearts, catheterization is indicated to: a. Assess the nature of pulmonary artery obstruction, with potential to restore maximal continuous, effective, unimpeded systemic venous flow to the maximal number of pulmonary artery segments. b. Assess and eliminate systemic–to–pulmonary vein collaterals. c. Assess and eliminate systemic–to–pulmonary artery connections. d. For adults with systemic–to–pulmonary shunts, the potential for perioperative transcatheter shunt exclusion should be examined.	I:C
Recommendation for Surgical Options for Patients With Single Ventricle	Surgeons with training and expertise in CHD should perform operations for single-ventricle anatomy or physiology.	I:C
Recommendation for Evaluation and Follow-Up After Fontan Procedure	Lifelong follow-up is recommended for patients after a Fontantype operation; this should include a yearly evaluation by a cardiologist with expertise in the care of ACHD patients.	I:C
Recommendation for Imaging	All patients with prior Fontan-type repair should have periodic echocardiographic and/or magnetic resonance examinations performed by staff with expertise in ACHD.	I:C
Recommendation for Diagnostic and Interventional Catheterization for Adults After Fontan Procedure	Catheterization of adults with a Fontan-type repair of singleventricle physiology should be performed in regional centers with expertise in ACHD.	I:C
Recommendations for Management Strategies for the Patient With Prior Fontan Repair	Management of patients with prior Fontan repair should be coordinated with a regional ACHD center. Local cardiologists, internists, and family care physicians should develop ongoing relationships with such a center with continuous availability of specialists.	I:C
	At least yearly follow-up is recommended for patients after Fontan repair.	I:C
	Arrhythmia management is frequently an issue, and consultation with an electrophysiologist is recommended as a vital part of care.	I:C
	New-onset atrial tachyarrhythmia should prompt a comprehensive noninvasive imaging evaluation to identify associated atrial/baffle thrombus, anatomic abnormalities of the Fontan pathway, or ventricular dysfunction.	I:C
Recommendations for Medical Therapy	Warfarin should be given for patients who have a documented atrial shunt, atrial thrombus, atrial arrhythmias, or a thromboembolic event.	I:C
	It is reasonable to treat SV dysfunction with ACE inhibitors and diuretics.	IIa:C
Recommendations for Surgery for Adults With Prior Fontan Repair	Surgeons with training and expertise in CHD should perform operations on patients with prior Fontan repair for singleventricle physiology.	I:C
	Reoperation after Fontan is indicated for the following: a. Unintended residual ASD that results in right-to-left shunt with symptoms and/or cyanosis not amenable to transcatheter closure. b. Hemodynamically significant residual systemic artery–to–pulmonary artery shunt, residual surgical shunt, or residual ventricle–to–pulmonary artery connection not amenable to transcatheter closure. c. Moderate to severe systemic AV valve regurgitation. d. Significant (greater than 30 mm Hg peak-to-peak) subaortic obstruction. e. Fontan pathway obstruction. f. Development of venous collateral channels or pulmonary arteriovenous malformation not amenable to transcatheter management. g. Pulmonary venous obstruction. h. Rhythm abnormalities, such as complete AV block or sick sinus syndrome, that require epicardial pacemaker insertion. i. Creation or closure of a fenestration not amenable to transcatheter intervention.	I:C
	Reoperation for Fontan conversion (ie, revision of an atriopulmonary connection to an intracardiac lateral tunnel, intra-atrial conduit, or extracardiac conduit) can be useful for recurrent atrial fibrillation or flutter without hemodynamically significant anatomic abnormalities. A concomitant Maze procedure should also be performed.	IIa:C
	Heart transplantation may be beneficial for severe SV dysfunction or protein-losing enteropathy.	IIb:C

(Table 21) Contd.....

	Recommendation	**Level of evidence**
Recommendations for Electrophysiology Testing/Pacing Issues in Single-Ventricle Physiology and After Fontan Procedure	Arrhythmia management is frequently an issue in patients after the Fontan procedure, and consultation with an electrophysiologist with expertise in CHD is recommended as a vital part of care.	I:C
	New-onset atrial tachyarrhythmias should prompt a comprehensive noninvasive imaging evaluation to identify associated atrial/baffle thrombus, anatomic abnormalities of the Fontan pathway, or ventricular dysfunction.	I:C
	Electrophysiological studies in adults with Fontan physiology should be performed at centers with expertise in the management of such patients.	I:C
	Clinicians must be mindful of the high risk for symptomatic IART in adult patients who have undergone the Fontan operation. This arrhythmia can cause serious hemodynamic compromise and contribute to atrial thrombus formation. Treatment is often difficult, and consultation with an electrophysiologist who is experienced with CHD is recommended whenever recurrent IART is detected.	I:C

REFERENCES

[1] Warnes CA, Liberthson R, Danielson GK, *et al.* Task force 1: the changing profile of congenital heart disease in adult life. J Am Coll Cardiol. 2001 ; 37: 1170-1175.

[2] Zipes DP, Libby P, Bonow R. Braunwald E. Braunwald's Heart Disease: A Textbook of Cardiovascular Medicine, 7th edition. New York: Elsevier Saunders; 2005: 1489-1552.

[3] Silka MJ, Hardy BG, Menashe VD, Morris CD. A population-based prospective evaluation of risk of sudden cardiac death after operation for common congenital heart defects. J Am Coll Cardiol, 1998; 32: 245-251.

[4] Concor registry. www.concor.net

[5] Dittmann H, Jacksch R, Voelker W, Karsch KR, Seipel L. Accuracy of Doppler echocardiography in quantification of left to right shunts in adult patients with atrial septal defects. J Am Coll Cardiol. 1988; 11: 338-342.

[6] Eren M, Dagderiren B, Bolca O. Proximal isovelocity surface area (PISA) as a non invasive method for the estimation if the shunt quantification in perimembraneous ventricular septal defects. Echocardiography 2001; 18: 137-147.

[7] Ueda Y, Hozumi T, Yoshida K, *et al.* Non invasive automated assessment of the ratio if pulmonary to systemic flow in patients with atrial septal defects by the color Doppler velocity profile integration method. Heart 2002; 88: 278-282.

[8] Hofmann T, Franzen O, Koschyk DH, Von Kodolitsch Y, Goldmann D, Meinertz T. Three-dimensional color Doppler echocardiography for assessing shunt volume in atrial septal defects. J Am Soc Echocardiogr. 2004; 17: 173-178.

[9] Mansencal N, Martin F, Farcot JC, *et al.* Echocardiographic automated cardiac output measurement of pulmonary output and quantification of intracardiac shunt. Int J Cardiol. 2005; 104: 25-31.

[10] Brenner LD, Caputo GR, Mostbeck G, *et al.* Quantification of left to right atrial shunts with velocity encoded cine nuclear magnetic resonance imaging. J Am Coll Cardiol. 1992; 20: 1246-1250.

[11] Hundley WG, Li HF, Lange RA, *et al.* Assessment of left to right intracardiac shunting by velocity encoded phase difference magnetic resonance imaging. A comparison with oximetric and indicator dilution techniques. Circulation 1995; 91: 2955-2960.

[12] Petersen SE, Voigtländer T, Kreitner KF, *et al.* Quantification of shunt volumes in congenital heart disease using a breath-hold MR phase contrast technique: comparison with oximetry. Int J Cardiovasc Imaging. 2002; 18: 53-60.

[13] Festa P, Ait-Ali L, Cerillo AG, De Marchi D, Murzi B. Magnetic resonance imaging is the diagnostic tool of choice in the preoperative evaluation of patients with partial anomalous pulmonary venous return. Int J Cardiovasc Imaging. 2006; 22: 685-93.

[14] Esmaeili A, Höhn R, Koch A, Vogl TJ, Hofstetter R, Abolmaali N. Assessment of shunt volumes in children with ventricular septal defects: comparative quantification of MR flow measurements and invasive oximetry. Clin Res Cardiol. 2006; 95: 523-530.

[15] Askenazi J, Ahnberg DS, Korngold E, LaFarge CG, Maltz DL, Treves S. Quantitative radionuclide angiocardiography: detection and quantification of left to right shunts. Am J Cardiol. 1976; 4: 382-387.

[16] Ham HR, Dobbeleir A, Virat P, Piepsz A, Lenaers A. Radionuclide quantitation of left-to right cardiac shunts using deconvolution analysis: concise communication. J Nucl Med. 1981; 22: 688-692.

[17] Kress P, Bitter F, Stauch M, *et al.* Radionuclide ventriculography: a non invasive method for the detection and quantification of left to right shunts in atrial septal defect. Clin Cardiol. 1982; 5: 192-200.

[18] Rigo P, Chevigné M. Measurement of left-to-right shunts by gated radionuclide angiography: concise communication. J Nucl Med. 1982; 23: 1070-1075.

[19] Anderson PA, Bowyer KW, Jones RH. Effects of age on radionuclide angiographic detection and quantification of left-to-right shunts. Am J Cardiol. 1984; 53: 879-83.

[20] Grossman W. Cardiac Catheterization, Angiography, and Intervention, 2nd edition. London: Henry Kimptom Publishers; 1980: 131-144.

[21] Oh JK, Seward JB, Tajik AJ. The Echo Manual, 3rd Edition. Philadelphia: Lippincott Williams & Wilkins; 2006: 332-367.

[22] Anderson B. Echocardiography: The Normal Examination and Echocardiographic Measurements, 2nd edition: MGA Graphics, 2007: 87-104

[23] Van Hare GF, Silverman NH. Contrast two-dimensional echocardiography in congenital heart disease: techniques, indications and clinical utility. J Am Coll Cardiol. 1989 Mar 1;13(3):673-86.

[24] Chang RK, Alejos JC, Atkinson D, *et al.* Bubble contrast echocardiography in detecting pulmonary arteriovenous shunting in children with univentricular heart after cavopulmonary anastomosis. J Am Coll Cardiol. 1999 Jun;33(7):2052-8.

[25] Kilner PJ, Gatehouse PD, Firmin DN. Flow measurement by magnetic resonance: a unique asset worth optimising. J Cardiovasc Magn Reson 2007; 9: 723-728

[26] Iskandrian AE, Verani MS (eds). Nuclear cardiac imaging: principles and Applications. 2nd Edition, F.A.Davis, 1996; 145-147.

[27] Wang ZJ, Reddy GP, Gotway MB, Yeh BM, Higgins CB. Cardiovascular shunts: MR imaging evaluation. RadioGraphics 2003; 23: S181–S194.

[28] Shub C, Dimopoulos IN, Seward JB, *et al.* Sensitivity of two dimensional echocardiography in the direct visualization of atrial septal defect utilizing the subcostal approach: experience with 154 patients. J Am Coll Cardiol. 1983; 2: 127-135.

[29] Minagoe S, Tei C, Kisanuki A, *et al.* Noninvasive pulsed Doppler echocardiographic detection of the direction of shunt flow in patients with atrial septal defect: usefulness of the right parasternal approach. Circulation. 1985; 7: 745-753.

[30] Hausmann D, Daniel WG, Mügge A, Ziemer G, Pearlman AS. Value of transesophageal color Doppler echocardiography for detection of different types of atrial septal defect in adults. J Am Soc Echocardiogr. 1992; 5: 481-488.

[31] Diethelm L, Déry R, Lipton MJ, Higgins CB. Atrial level shunts: Sensitivity and specificity of MR diagnosis. Radiology 1987; 162: 181-86

[32] Pascoe RD, Oh JK, Warnes CA, Danielson GK, Tajik AJ, Seward JB. Diagnosis of Sinus Venosus Atrial Septal Defect With Transesophageal Echocardiography. Circulation 1996; 94: 1049-1055.

[33] Roberson DA, Muhiudeen IA, Silverman NH, Turley K, Haas GS, Cahalan MK. Intraoperative transesophageal echocardiography of atrioventricular septal defect. J Am Coll Cardiol. 1991; 18: 537-45.

[34] Valente AM, Sena L, Powell AJ, Del Nido PJ, Geva T. Cardiac Magnetic Resonance Imaging Evaluation of Sinus Venosus Defects. Pediatric Cardiol. 2007; 28: 51-56

[35] Otterstad JE, Simonsen S, Vatne K, Myhre E. Doppler echocardiography in adults with isolated ventricular septal defect. Eur Heart J. 1984; 5: 332-337

[36] Sree Ram MN, Sreedhar CM, Akam A, Indrajit IK. The role of cardiac MRI in congenital heart disease. Chest 2005; 15: 239-246.

[37] Shyu KG, Lai LP, Lin SC, Chang H, Chen JJ. Diagnostic accuracy of transesophageal echocardiography for detecting patent ductus arteriosus in adolescent and adults. Chest 1995; 108: 1201-1205.

[38] Hartnell GG, Cohen MC, Meier RA, Finn JP. Magnetic resonance angiography demonstration of congenital heart disease in adults. Clin Radiol. 1996; 51: 851-857.

[39] Houston A, Hillis S, Lilley S, Richens T, Swan L. Echocardiography in adult congenital heart disease. Heart 1998; 80: S12-S26.

[40] Jenni R, Vieli A. PDA by Doppler echo. Circulation. 1980; 61: 865.-866.

[41] Marx GR, Fulton DR, Pandian NG, *et al.* Delineation of site, relative size and dynamic geometry of atrial septal defects by real time three dimensional echocardiography. J Am Coll Cardiol. 1995; 25: 482-490.

[42] Pollick C, Sullivan H, Cujec B, Wilansky S. Doppler color flow imaging assessment of shunt size in atrial size defect. Circulation 1988; 78: 522-528.

[43] Lange A, Walayat M, Turnbull CM, *et al.* Assessment of atrial septal defect morphology by transthoracic three dimensional echocardiography using standard gray and Doppler myocardial imaging techniques: Comparison with magnetic resonance imaging and intraoperative findings. Heart 1997; 78: 382-389.

[44] Zhu W, Cao QL, Rhodes J, Hijazi ZM. Measurement of atrial septal defect size: A comparative study between three-dimensional transesophageal echocardiography and the standard balloon sizing method. Pediatric Cardiol. 2000; 21: 465-469.

[45] Koenig P, Cao QL, Heitschmidt M, Waight DJ, Hijazi ZM. Role of intracardiac echocardiographic guidance in transcatheter closure of atrial septal defects and patent foramen ovale using the Amplatzer device. J Interv Cardiol. 2003; 16: 51-62.

[46] Mehmood F, Vengala S, Nanda NC, *et al.* Usefulness of live Three Dimensional Transthoracic Echocardiography in the Characterization of Atrial Septal defects in Adults. Echocardiography 2004; 21: 707-713

[47] Durongpisitkul K, Tang NL, Soongswang J, Laohaprasitiporn D, Nanal A. Predictors of Successful Transcatheter Closure of Atrial Septal Defect by Cardiac Magnetic Resonance Imaging. Pediatric Cardiol. 2004; 25: 124-130.

[48] Chen FL, Hsiung MC, Hsieh KS, Li YC, Chou MC. Real time three dimensional transthoracic echocardiography for guiding Amplatzer Septal Occluder device deployment in patients with atrial septal defect. Echocardiography 2006; 23: 763-770.

[49] Rigatelli G, Cardaioli P, Braggion G, *et al.* Transesophageal echocardiography and intracardiac echocardiography differently predict potential technical challenges or failures of interatrial shunts catheter-based closure. J Interv Cardiol. 2007; 20: 77-81.

[50] Holmvang G, Palacios IF, Vlahakes GJ, *et al.* Imaging and sizing of atrial septal defects by magnetic resonance. Circulation 1995; 92: 3473-3480.

[51] Thomson LE, Crowley AL, Heitner JF, *et al.* Direct En Face Imaging of Secundum Atrial Septal Defects by Velocity-Encoded Cardiovascular Magnetic Resonance in Patients Evaluated for Possible Transcatheter Closure. Circ Cardiovasc Imaging. 2008; 1: 31 - 40.

[52] Weber C, Weber M, Ekinci O, *et al.* Atrial septal defects type II: noninvasive evaluation of patients before implantation of an Amplatzer Septal Occluder and on follow-up by magnetic resonance imaging compared with TEE and invasive measurement. Eur Radiol. 2008 [Epub ahead of print].

[53] Cao QL, Zabal C, Koenig P, Sandhu S, Hijazi ZM. Initial clinical experience with intracadiac echocardiography in guiding transcatheter closure of perimembranous ventricular septal defects: feasibility and comparison with transesophageal echocardiography. Catheter Cardiovasc Interv. 2005; 66: 258-267.

[54] Van den Bosch AE, Ten Harkel DJ, McGhie JS, *et al.* Characterization of atrial septal defect assessed by real-time 3 dimensional echocardiography. J Am Soc Echocardiogr. 2006; 19: 815-821.

[55] Douglas PS, Khandheria B, Stainback RF, *et al.* 2007 Appropriateness criteria for transthoracic and transesophageal echocardiography. J Am Coll Cardiol. 2007; 50: 187-204.

[56] Hendel RC, Patel MR, Kramer CM, *et al.* 2006 appropriateness criteria for cardiac computed tomography and cardiac magnetic resonance imaging. J Am Coll Cardiol. 2006; 48: 1475-1497.

[57] Inglessis I, Landzberg M. Interventional catheterization in Adult Congenital Heart Disease. Circulation 2007; 115: 1622-1633.

[58] Warnes CA, Williams RG, Bashore TM, *et al*; American College of Cardiology; American Heart Association Task Force on Practice Guidelines (Writing Committee to Develop Guidelines on the Management of Adults With Congenital Heart Disease); American Society of Echocardiography; Heart Rhythm Society; International Society for Adult Congenital Heart Disease; Society for Cardiovascular Angiography and Interventions; Society of Thoracic Surgeons. ACC/AHA 2008 guidelines for the management of adults with congenital heart disease: a report of the American College of Cardiology/American Heart Association Task Force on Practice Guidelines (Writing Committee to Develop Guidelines on the Management of Adults With Congenital Heart Disease). Developed in Collaboration With the American Society of Echocardiography, Heart Rhythm Society, International Society for Adult Congenital Heart Disease, Society for Cardiovascular Angiography and Interventions, and Society of Thoracic Surgeons. J Am Coll Cardiol. 2008; 52: e1-121.

[59] Omeish A, Hijazi Z. Transcatheter closure of atrial septal defect in children and adults using the Amplatz septal occluder. J Interven Cardiol. 2001; 14: 37-44.

[60] Earing MG, Cabalka AK, Seward JB, Bruce CJ, Reeder GS, Hagler DJ. Intracardiac echocardiographic guidance during transcatheter device closure of atrial septal defect and patent foramen ovale. May Clin Proc. 2004; 79: 24-34.

[61] Ammash N, Warnes C. Ventricular septal defect in Adults. Ann Intern Med. 2001; 135: 812-824.

[62] Carminati M, Butera G, Chessa M, *et al*; Investigators of the European VSD Registry. Transcatheter closure of congenital ventricular septal defects: results of the European Registry. Eur Heart J. 2007; 28: 2361-2368.

[63] Butera G, Chessa M, Carminati M. Percutaneous closure of ventricular septal defects. State of the art. J Cardiovasc Med. 2007; 8: 39-45.

[64] Butera G, Carminati M, Chessa M, *et al.* Transcatheter closure of perimembraneous ventricular septal defects. J Am Coll Cardiol. 2007; 50: 1189-1195

[65] Lee CH, Leung YL, Kwong NP, Kwok OH, Yip AS, Chow WH. Transcatheter closure of patent ductus arteriosus in Chinese adults: immediate and long-term results. J Invasive Cardiol. 2003; 15: 26-30.

[66] Aboulhoson J, Child J. Left ventricular outflow obstruction: Subaortic stenosis, bicuspid aortic valve, supravalvular aortic stenosis, and coarctation of the aorta. Circulation 2006; 114: 2412-2422.

[67] Roche KJ, Genieser NB, Ambrosino MM, Henry GL. MR findings in Shone's complex of left heart obstructive lesions. Pediatr Radiol 1998 28:841-5.

[68] Modi KA, Annamali S, Ernest K, Pratep CR. Diagnosis and surgical correction of cor triatriatum in an adult: Combined use of transesophageal and contrast echocardiography, and a review of literature. Echocardiography 2006; 23: 506-509.

[69] Agrawal GG, Nanda NC, Htay T, Dod HS, Gandhari SR. Live three-dimensional transthoracic echocardiographic identification of discrete subaortic membranous stenosis. Echocardiography 2003; 20: 617-619

[70] Task Force Report. The clinical role of magnetic resonance in cardiovascular disease. Eur Heart J. 1998; 19: 19-39.

[71] Brickner E, Hillis D, and Lange R. Congenital heart disease in Adults: First of two parts. N Engl J Med. 2000; 342: 256-263.

[72] Didier D, Saint-Martin C, Lapierre C, *et al.* Coarctation of the aorta: pre and postoperative evaluation with MRI and MR angiography; correlation with echocardiography and surgery. Int J Cardiovas Imaging 2006; 22: 457-475.

[73] McCrindle B. Coarctation of the aorta. Current Opinion in Cardiology 1999; 14: 448-454.

[74] Kinsara A, Chan KL. Non invasive imaging modalities in coarctation of the aorta. Chest 2004; 126: 1016-1018.

[75] Tan JL, Babu-Narayan SV, Henein MY, Mullen M, Li W. Doppler echocardiography profile and indexes in the evaluation of aortic coarctation in patients before and after stenting. J Am Coll Card. 2005; 46: 1045-1053.

[76] Riquelme C, Laissy JP, Menegazzo D, *et al.* MR imaging of coarctation of the aorta and its postoperative complications in adults: assessment with spin echo and cine-MRI. Magn Reson Imaging 1999; 17: 37-46.

[77] Godart F, Labrot G, Devos P, McFadden E, Rey C, Beregi JP. Coarctation of the aorta: comparison of aortic dimensions between conventional MR imaging, 3D MR angiography, and conventional angiography. Eur Radiol. 2002; 12: 2034-2039.

[78] Gutberlet M, Hosten N, Vogel M, *et al.* Quantification of morphologic and hemodynamic severity of coarctation of the aorta by magnetic resonance imaging. Cardiol Young. 2001; 11: 512-520.

[79] Hom J, Ordovas K, and Redy G. Velocity-encoded Cine MR imaging in aortic coarctation: Functional assessment of hemodynamic events. Radiographics 2008; 28: 407-416.

[80] Nielsen JC, Powell AJ, Gauvreau K, Marcus EN, Prakash A, Geva T. Magnetic resonance imaging predictors of coarctation severity. Circulation 2005; 111: 622-628.

[81] Hager A, Kaemmerer H, Leppert A, *et al.* Follow-up of adults with coarctation of the aorta: comparison of helical CT and MRI, and impact on assessing diameter changes. Chest. 2004;126:1169-1176.

[82] Rodés-Cabau J, Miró J, Dancea A, *et al.* Comparison of surgical and transcatheter treatment for native coarctation of the aorta in patients > or = 1 year old. The Quebec Native Coarctation of the Aorta study. Am Heart J. 2007; 154: 186-92

[83] Brickner E, Hillis D, Lange R. Congenital heart disease in Adults: Second of two parts. New Engl J Med. 2000; 342: 334-342.

[84] Yetman AT, Graham T. The dilated aorta in patients with congenital cardiac defects. J Am Coll Cardiol. 2009;53:461-7.

[85] Boechat MI, Ratib O, Williams PL, Gomes AS, Child JS, Allada V. Cardiac MRI imaging and MR angiography for assessment of complex Tetralogy of Fallot and pulmonary atresia. Radiographics 2005; 25: 1535-1546.

[86] Boernemeier R, Weinberg P, Fogel M. Angiographic, echocardiographic, and three-dimensional magnetic resonance imaging of extracardiac conduits in congenital heart disease. Am J Cardiol. 1996; 78: 713-717.

[87] Oosterhof T, van Straten A, Vliegen HW, *et al.* Preoperative Thresholds for Pulmonary Valve Replacement in Patients With Corrected Tetralogy of Fallot Using Cardiovascular Magnetic Resonance. Circulation. 2007; 116: 545 - 551.

[88] Wang XM, Wu LB, Sun C, *et al.* Clinical application of 64 slice spiral CT in the diagnosis of the Tetralogy of Fallot. Eur J Radiol. 2007; 64: 296-301.

[89] Warnes C. Transposition of the Great arteries. Circulation 2006; 114: 2699-2709.

[90] Ahmed S, Nekkanti R, Nanda NC, Yousif AM. Three dimensional transesophageal echocardiographic demonstration of interaatrial baffle obstruction. Echocardiography 2003; 20: 683-686.

[91] Oosterhof T, Mulder BJ, Vliegen HW, de Roos A. Cardiovascular magnetic resonance in the follow up of patients with corrected Tetralogy of Fallot: A review. Am Heart J. 2006; 151: 265-272.

[92] Fogel M, Hubbard A, Weinberg P. A simplified approach for assessment of intracardiac baffles and extracardiac conduits in congenital heart surgery with two and three dimensional magnetic resonance imaging. Am Heart J. 2001; 142: 1028-1036.

[93] Reiter G, Reiter U, Kovasc G, *et al.* Magnetic Resonance–Derived 3-Dimensional Blood Flow Patterns in the Main Pulmonary Artery as a Marker of Pulmonary Hypertension and a Measure of Elevated Mean Pulmonary Arterial Pressure. Circ Cardiovasc Imaging. 2008; 1: 23 - 30.

[94] Warnes C, Somerville J. Tricuspid atresia in adolescents and adults: current state and late complications. Heart 1986; 56: 535-543.

[95] Coon PD, Rychik J, Novello RT, Ro PS, Gaynor JW, Spray TL. Thrombus formation after the Fontan operation. Ann Thorac Surg. 2001; 71: 1990-1994.

[96] Tsang W, Johansson B, Salehian O, Holm J, Webb G, Gatzoulis MA, Therrien J. Intracardiac thrombus in adults with the Fontan circulation. Cardiol Young. 2007; 17: 646-51.

[97] Goo HW, Yang DH, Park IS, *et al.* Time resolved three dimensional contrast enhanced magnetic resonance angiography in patients who have undergone a Fontan operation or bidirectional cavopulmonary connection: initial experience. J Magn Reson Imaging. 2007; 25: 727-736.

[98] Takawira F, Ayer JG, Onikul E, *et al.* Evaluation of the extracardiac conduit modification of the Fontan operation for thrombus formation using magnetic resonance imaging. Heart Lung Circ. 2008; 17: 407-10.

[99] Casolo G, Rega L, Gensini GF. Detection of right atrial and pulmonary artery thrombosis after the Fontan procedure by magnetic resonance imaging. Heart. 200; 90: 825

[100] Ammash NM, Warnes CA, Connolly HM, Danielson GK, Seward JB. Mimics of Ebstein's anomaly. Am Heart J 1997; 134: 508-513.

[101] Patel V, Nanda NC, Rajdev S, *et al.* Live/real time three dimensional transthoracic echocardiographic assessment of Ebstein's anomaly. Echocardiography 2005; 22: 847-854.

[102] Gurvitz M, Stout K. Ebstein's anomaly of the tricuspid valve. Curr Cardiol Rep. 2007; 9: 336-42.

[103] McConnell MV, Ganz P, Selwyn AP, Li W, Edelman RR, Manning WJ. Identification of anamolous coronary arteries and their anatomic course by magnetic resonance coronary angiography. Circulation 1995; 92: 3158-3162.

[104] Taylor AM, Thorne SA, Rubens MB, *et al.* Coronary artery imaging in grown up congenital heart disease: complementary role of magnetic resonance and x-ray coronary angiography. Circulation 2000; 101: 1670-1678.

[105] Schmitt R, Froehner S, Brunn J, *et al.* Congenital anomalies of the coronary arteries: imaging with contrast-enhanced, multidetector computed tomography. Eur Radiol 2005; 15: 1110-1121.

[106] Kim SY, Seo JB, Do KH, *et al.* Coronary artery anomalies: classification and ECG-gated multi-detector row CT findings with angiographic correlation. Radiographic 2006; 26: 317-334.

[107] Schmid M, Achenbach S, Ludwig J, *et al.* Visualization of coronary artery anomalies by contrast enhanced multi-detector row spiral computed tomography. Int J Cardiol. 2006; 111: 430-443.

[108] Angelini P and Flamm S. Newer concepts for imaging anomalous aortic origin of the coronary arteries in adults. Cath and Cardiov Interv. 2007; 69: 942-954.

[109] Giannoccaro PJ, Sochowski RA, Morton BC, Chan KL. Complementary role of transesophageal echocardiography to coronary angiography in the assessment of coronary anomalies. Heart 1993; 70: 70-74.

[110] Fernandes F, Alam M, Smith S, Khaja F. The role of transesophageal echocardiography in identifying anomalous coronary arteries. Circulation 1993; 88: 2532-2540.

[111] Ilgenli TF, Nanda NC, Sinha A, Khanna D. Live three dimensional transthoracic echocardiographic assessment of anomalous origin of left coronary artery from the pulmonary artery. Echocardiography 2004; 21: 559-562.

[112] Welker M, Salanitri J, Deshpande VS, Shea SM, Li D, Pereles FS. Coronary artery anomalies diagnosed by magnetic resonance angiography. Australian Radiology 2006; 50: 114-121.

[113] Ishikawa T, Brandt PW. Anomalous origin of the left main coronary artery from the right anterior aortic sinus: angiographic definition of anomalous course. Am J Cardiol. 1985; 55: 770-776.

[114] Angelini P, Velasco JA, Ott D, Khoshnevis GR. Anomalous coronary artery arising from the opposite sinus: descriptive features and pathophysiologic mechanisms, as documented by intravascular ultrasonography. J Invasive Cardiol. 2003; 15: 507-14.

[115] Mintz GS, Iskandrian AS, Bemis CE, Mundth ED, Owens JS. Myocardial ischemia in anomalous origin of the right coronary artery from the pulmonary trunk. Proof of a coronary steal. Am J Cardiol. 1983; 51: 610-612.

[116] Finley JP, Howman-Giles R, Gilday DL, Olley PM, Rowe RD. Thallium-201 myocardial imaging in anomalous left coronary artery arising from the pulmonary artery. Applications before and after medical and surgical treatment. Am J Cardiol. 1978; 42: 675-680.

[117] Brenner DJ, Hall EJ. Computed tomography-an increasing source of radiation exposure. N Engl J Med. 2007; 357: 277-84.

[118] Kallen AJ, Jhung MA, Cheng S, *et al.* Gadolinium-containing magnetic resonance imaging contrast and nephrogenic systemic fibrosis: a case-control study. Am J Kidney Dis. 2008;51: 966-75.

Keyword/Subject Index

Printed in Dunstable, United Kingdom

91335490R00047